Tried and True

Tried and True

✦

Skin Care Products, Techniques and Procedures that will Revitalize and Restore over 40 Skin

by
Catherine Clarke

iUniverse, Inc.
New York Lincoln Shanghai

Tried and True
Skin Care Products, Techniques and Procedures that will Revitalize and Restore over 40 Skin

iUniverse books may be ordered through booksellers or by contacting:

iUniverse
2021 Pine Lake Road, Suite 100
Lincoln, NE 68512
www.iuniverse.com
1-800-Authors (1-800-288-4677)

The intent of this book is to inform the consumer. Please consult with a health care professional, if needed, before purchasing any new skin care products especially if you have sensitive skin.

ISBN-13: 978-0-595-37327-7 (pbk)
ISBN-13: 978-0-595-81725-2 (ebk)
ISBN-10: 0-595-37327-5 (pbk)
ISBN-10: 0-595-81725-4 (ebk)

Printed in the United States of America

Contents

Introduction..ix

CHAPTER 1   What is Your Skin Going to
Eat and Drink Today?.........................1

CHAPTER 2   What is Skin? 4

CHAPTER 3   Face, Neck and Eye Toning and
Beneficial Enhancing Devices 8

CHAPTER 4   Scraping Off the Top Layer
Removing Makeup..............................16

CHAPTER 5   Away With the Grime
Cleansers 18

CHAPTER 6   Tone Your Body/Tone Your Skin
Toners, Astringents and Clarifiers................31

CHAPTER 7   Scrubbing Off the Years
Exfoliators 46

CHAPTER 8   Vitamins In, Vitamins Out
Vitamins and Serums 58

CHAPTER 9   Invisible Protective Barrier
Moisturizers 72

CHAPTER 10   Lifting Up the Years
Lifting and Firming 86

CHAPTER 11   Procedures 117

CHAPTER 12   Spa Treatment 128

CHAPTER 13   Homemade Skin Care
Recipes...135

CHAPTER 14   Must Buy Kits 177

CHAPTER 15   Conclusion..197

Contact Information...207

Credits 209

Alphabetical Order Beauty Enhancing Devices 211

About the Author 213

Acknowledgement

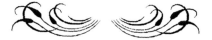

I would like to thank my four children, Jimmy, Kitty, Michael and Theresa for all their support, encouragement and unshakable confidence for which they have shown me. Thank you for your joy, laughter and most of all love.

Introduction

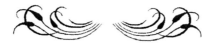

Congratulations! You have just taken the first step toward a more youthful appearance. Within this book you will find techniques, procedures and an extensive collection of skin care products that will repair and restore your skin, thus reversing the visible signs of aging.

I have saved you time and money by purchasing and testing the many skin care products mentioned in this book. You too can experience a more natural, healthy, glowing and youthful appearance just by purchasing skin care products that do exactly what the manufacturer has advertised. The skin care products in this book will give you a more youthful appearance.

When purchasing skin care products it is important that the products you select perform as promised. If that product does not perform as advertised you have not only wasted your time but you have also wasted your money. All the skin care products within this book will give you the results that the manufacturer claims.

You should select skin care products that are age appropriate. If you are over 40, you should not be using the same skin care products that you were using in your 20's and 30's. There are skin care products for women over the age of 40 that will repair discolored, lined, wrinkled and sagging skin and those products are in this book.

Always keep in mind that your fine lines and wrinkles did not appear overnight and they will not disappear overnight. Please also keep in mind there are different skin types and that issue must be addressed when selecting new skin care products.

Some products and procedures that I mention will give you instant but temporary results while others, and I will call them treatments, will work over a period of time.

Finding the right type of skin care products for your particular skin type can be accomplished by going to a professional. That professional will look at the condition of your skin and by a series of questions, will be able to tell you what skin type you have and exactly what condition your skin is in and then you will be ready to purchase the skin care products for your skin's needs.

When you have selected a skin care product be consistent giving it time, approximately four to eight weeks, to repair and restore your skin. The end result of your skin renewing process will depend on the condition of your skin and how dedicated you are toward getting older gracefully. The more fine lines and wrinkles you have, the longer it will take to minimize them but it can do done.

There are remarkable products for over 40 pre-menopausal or menopausal skin on the market today that will help you achieve a healthier, radiant, more youthful appearance. Over 40 skin does need special attention when selecting new skin care products. Between the ages of 35 and 40 is when you start seeing the outward signs of aging. Life style as well as genetics will determine a person's physical appearance.

Within the past ten years, family members and I have tested all the skin care products in this book and have found them to be effective for one reason or another. I have also had a few procedures performed at a dermatologist's office that did minimize my fine lines and wrinkles while giving me a more youthful appearance.

The techniques that I reference and recommend are almost effortless and the products are "Tried and True." Yes, they do work.

There is another reason I have written this book and that reason is the cost of skin care products. More often than not, that cost can be exorbitant; I have found skin care products that are affordable while achieving remarkable results. Approximately 98% of the skin care products in this book have a 30-day money-back guarantee and for that reason, you can experiment with peace of mind. When a manufacturer has enough confidence in their products to give you a money-back guarantee, then so can you.

Today is the day that you will start your transformation back in time. You can transform your skin by using skin care products made for a specific purpose and that purpose is to repair and restore your skin giving you a more youthful and healthy appearance.

I would like to emphasize two very important steps before you continue further. The two steps that I would like to emphasize are: you must exfoliate and hydrate your skin.

When you exfoliate your skin you are getting rid of the old dead skin cells that have accumulated over a period of years. That accumulation of dead skin cells is the reason your skin is lined, wrinkled and discolored.

The reason you should hydrate your skin is to plump up your skin with moisturizing ingredients and that hydration will minimize the appearance of your lines and wrinkles.

You must choose the best skin care products for your particular skin type and condition, no matter what skin type you have those products are in this book. The condition that your skin is in will be significant when selecting new skin care products. It is the loss of collagen and elastin that create your fine lines and wrinkles. One way to address these aging issues is to select skin care products with anti-aging ingredients which will rejuvenate, restore and revitalize aging, mature skin.

Just by looking into a mirror, you can see exactly what problems you should address. When you look into a mirror, look for skin discoloration, fine lines and wrinkles. If you are at the age where your skin is beginning to sag, that is another issued that must be addressed. Whatever your skin's needs are, you can address them with skin care products with anti-aging ingredients. Write down the results you would like to achieve. Buy your products based on your particular issues. If you are consistent, you will be amazed at your results.

This book has chapters and in each chapter there are skin care products that will give you the maximum anti-aging results you are looking for. You will never waste your time or money again.

Cosmetic surgery is another option to reverse the aging process. If you want cosmetic surgery have the surgery the decision is yours. If you choose to grow older gracefully that's fine too. Whatever you decide, your skin must be in the best possible condition that it can be.

Your skin will have that youthful glow it once had just by removing the accumulated dead skin cells and using quality skin care products and those quality skin care products are in this book. From toning and firming your facial muscles, selecting the best exfoliation products, cleansers and toners to selecting the perfect vitamins and serums, yes, they are all within the pages of this book.

You can look as young as you feel and I can tell you honestly that before I started using anti-aging skin care products that I looked my age. Approximately six months after using anti-aging skin care products, I looked as young as I felt and so can you.

I want all women to feel and look as good as they can because women are the care givers. Most women do not take the time that they need to pamper themselves and they should. Before you know it you are 50 and the question is, "Do you want to look 50? Ladies it is time that you get started taking care of yourself for a change, you are worth it.

You only need 15 to 20 minutes a day to take proper care of your skin. The question is do you want to start looking younger? There are seven signs of aging that should be addressed and they are: uneven skin tone, uneven texture, lines & wrinkles, pore size, age spots, dryness and lackluster skin. When you purchase the best possible skin care products for your particular skin type, you will see the signs of aging slowly disappear.

Each and every skin care product in this book contains anti-aging ingredients. I will give you the name of the skin care product and then I will describe exactly how each skin care product will perform and at the end of the description I will inform you as to where each product can be purchased. The process is easy. I will give you the name of the product, what it does for your skin and where you can purchase the product, it is that simple. Now get started on your anti-aging journey.

1

What is Your Skin Going to Eat and Drink Today?

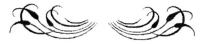

The title says it all. What you eat or drink today not only fuels your mind and body but your skin. The next time someone says to you, "You are what you eat" that person will be correct.

There are so many issues to take into consideration for a healthier more youthful appearance. What you eat and drink will play a significant role not only in the way you feel but also in the way you look.

It is important to start eating a healthy well-balanced diet at a very young age so that your skin will look and feel younger as you age. You can enhance the appearance of your skin by eating a well balanced diet. Just by eating a healthy balance of fruits and vegetables, meat, fish, chicken and fish, etc. your skin will not only look healthy but it will be healthy. Eating a proper diet should become part of your new beauty regimen.

Also remember to drink plenty of water, at least eight, eight-ounce glasses of water per day. It is a well-known fact that hydration is not only healthy for the inside but also for the outside. Hydrating your skin means that you will have fewer lines and wrinkles while flushing out toxins from your skin. Women, as a rule do not drink enough water. Drinking water must become a very important part of your beauty routine. Approximately 70% of our body is made up of water. When you deprive your body of water, hydration, you deprive your skin of the nutrients needed for a healthy glowing outward appearance. Drink plenty of water.

Eating the right types of food which contain the proper amount of vitamins and minerals, taking vitamin supplements and using quality skin care products that also contain vitamins which will assist your body's largest organ, your skin, in obtaining a more youthful appearance.

Vitamin C helps collagen formation which can maintain a plumper and younger looking skin. Vitamin A will protect your skin from the sun's harmful UV rays. Vitamin B12 can help firm the skin. Just remember back when you were very little and your mother said, "Eat you vegetable and fruit", mothers knew best. For a more youthful appearance eat plenty of fruits and vegetables, they are full of vitamins.

Sugar is very damaging and aging to the skin. Sugar can attach itself to collagen thus making the skin nonflexible.

Losing the reduction of elasticity in young skin will result in giving you more lines and deeper wrinkles as you age.

When you have an opportunity, log onto the internet or go to the library and look up, "Exactly what foods you eat that convert into sugar." You will be surprised.

Eating fish will add luster and softness to your skin. Eating vegetable and nuts will also promote great looking healthy skin. Low fat yogurt is also good for the skin. Berries, blueberries, strawberries & blackberries are loaded with antioxidants because they contain natural vitamins and antioxidants which do play a significant role in a healthier and more youthful appearance.

Your appearance is up to you. What you ingest, your life style and heredity, they all play a significant role in the way you look and feel. After the age of 40 adding skin care products that contain anti-aging ingredients is essential if you wish to age gracefully. At the age of 50 you can look 40 if you pay attention to all aspects of your daily routine.

Actually it is quite simple the foods that are healthy for you will also give you a younger looking appearance. If you are unaware of what foods you should be eating, go to a nutritionist, ask you family doctor, go onto the internet, well what are you waiting for? Eat healthy and look younger, what a combination.

2

What is Skin?

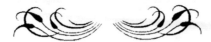

Your skin is a membrane and that membrane can be repaired and restored, therefore, reversing the signs of aging.

The skin is the largest organ in your body. Your skin has three layers and all three layers do their own job. The three layers of skin are the epidermis, dermis and subcutaneous fat. At the bottom of the epidermis, new skin cells are forming trying to rid your body of the old dead skin cell so that the new ones can replace them. The second layer is the dermis and the dermis accommodates your oil glands and that oil protects your skin. The third layer is the subcutaneous fat layer. The subcutaneous fat layer helps hold your skin to your tissues. Most of your facial muscles are attached to your skin.

The most common skin types are: normal, dry, oily & combination. It is important to know exactly what type skin you have. If you are not sure of your skin type, please go to the dermatologist, he or she will tell you your skin type and the condition of your skin.

There are two factors when determining the best possible skin care products and they are your skin type and the condition of your skin. You must know both before select any new skin care product purchases. There are quite a few questions you should ask yourself when determining new products and some of them are: Are you going through menopause? Do you smoke? Are you taking any medication? What is your daily exposure to the elements? I have mentioned just a few questions that will determine the purchase of any new skin care products.

You can have oily or combination skin that needs to be hydrated. You can have dry skin that needs exfoliating. So remember you need to know your skin type and the condition of your skin. As I stated earlier there are two factors to consider before selecting anti-aging skin care products skin type and condition. Both factors must be determined before applying skin care products.

I would like to mention just a few points of interest as to my morning routine. When I get up, I start by washing my face with a facial cleanser and I finish with a toner. After the washing process, I put on four serums and I only use one drop per serum. After my serums I put on my moisturizer but just a pea size and it is a hydrating moisturizer and to finish, I put on a good sunscreen.

I know that sound like a lot but it isn't. The serums that I use are: Vitamin C, Vitamin A, lifting serum and a hydrating serum but as I said earlier just one drop of each all over my entire face and neck. Then I will put a pea size drop of the hydrating cream on my face and to finish the face, I finalize the process with a pea size drop of the sunscreen. Then I will apply my neck cream and eye cream. I use so little that my skin care products do last a long time.

Most women use more then they should. You just need one drop of serum and a very small amount of moisturizer. I work in an office so my sunscreen is 15 and on the weekend if I am out-and-about I will use a 30 to 45 sunscreen. But remember sun is good in moderation. Everyone needs the sun for healthy bones.

Over the age of 40 you have to work at what once came naturally but the end result can be very rewarding.

Skin care products should be applied from the lightest to the heaviest consistency and that succession is as follows:

1.   Serums and/or vitamins

2.   Gels

3.   Lotions

4.   Creams

5.   Temporary lifting and/or firming products

If all else fails and you can not remember what goes on first, just remember to apply the thinnest product first and ending the process with your firming product unless otherwise directed by the manufacturer.

3

Face, Neck and Eye Toning and Beneficial Enhancing Devices

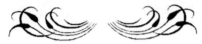

The first step in the restoration process is to firm and tone the face, eye and neck muscles. After the age of 30, your skin's collagen and elasticity begins to diminish and if that isn't enough, your facial muscles start to atrophy (droop) diminishing that firm and toned appearance it once had.

We have 57 facial muscles that flatten while gravity is pulling them down causing the facial muscles to elongate and eventually that process will change your facial structure.

Before starting your facial toning program, take a picture so that you can compare your before and after results.

You can tone and tighten your facial muscles just by exercising them giving your face, eye and neck areas a more youthful and toned appearance.

Your facial structure relies on firm facial muscles and in order for these muscles to be firm and toned, they need to be exercised. In most cases, your facial muscles are attached to your skin. So, therefore, when your facial muscles begin to atrophy, your skin begins to elongate or sag thus changing the entire structure of your face. Just like exercising your body, facial exercises must be performed regularly in order to keep that toned firm appearance.

Instead of exercising your facial muscles manually, why not let a machine do the exercises for you. When you are performing facial exercises manually, there is a possibility that you may do the exercises incorrectly but if you use a machine the probability is very minimal to none.

The facial muscle toning devices I use are as follows:

1) **Rejuvenique Facial Mask Toner**

    Customer Service: 1-800-934-7455 or Product Ordering 1-800-543-5427 or (www.rejuvenique.com)

The Rejuvenique Facial Mask Toner toning system consists of a facial mask with a number of contact points that deliver a light energy pulsation to key areas on your face and eye areas. After using this machine, the muscles on your face and around your eye area will start to lift and tighten resulting in a more toned appearance.

The more toned your facial muscles are the more lifted your skin becomes. When your skin becomes lifted there will be a reduction in your fine lines and wrinkles.

When you have completed the allotted time period the machine will automatically stop. I use this machine every other day.

2)   Hand Held Facial Toner Devices

This type of product can be found on the Internet or ask your favorite salon or beauty supplier.

A hand held facial toning device will tone your face, eye and neck areas. This toning device is a hand-held device that will exercise all the muscle groups. When your facial muscles become firm your fine lines and wrinkles will be diminished because you have lifted your sagging skin giving your face a more toned appearance.

If you want to work extra hard on one area after the specified routine, just do so. I use a hand held facial firming machine on the days that I do not use the Rejuvenique Facial Mask Toner.

Both of the facial muscle toning machines firm and tighten your facial muscles giving you a more youthful appearance.

3)   Facial Flex Ultra

www.biof.com/facialflex.html
The above listed website is where you may obtain additional information regarding the Facial Flex machine information.

The Facial-Flex Ultra is used by placing it into the corners of your mouth, then compressing and releasing, receptively, against the force of an elastic band. Performing these repetitive movements with Facial-Flex Ultra exercises the muscles of your face, chin and neck, against dynamic, constant, external resistance. Facial-Flex Ultra has been clinically proven to be effective in significantly increasing facial muscles strength, uplifting, contouring and firming the face in individuals exhibiting the effects of facial aging due to weakened facial muscles.

The results of this clinical testing facial firming device have been published by both the Society of Investigative Dermatology and in the Journal of Geriatric Dermatology. The Facial-Flex Ultra system emphasizes the importance of your entire face, chin and neck and the interdependence of the muscles, skin and interconnecting tissue.

I use this product every day for four minutes a day, because I have a jaw line and neck sagging problem.

Neck Area

Exercising your facial muscles is a very important part of your new beauty regimen. While most women do realize that exercising their facial muscles is important, they do not realize how important it is to exercise their neck muscles. The skin on the neck is different (thinner) and less porous from the skin on the face and will show the signs of aging much faster. You must tone and tighten your neck muscles for a complete overall toned look.

The easiest way I have found that specifically exercises the neck area is:

4)   Profile Toner (found on the internet)

This device will tone your jowl and neck areas. By using the Profile Toner your neck muscles will be more toned and contoured. When you exercise your neck area you will tighten the sagging skin and/or double chin. Lifting and smoothing the neck area will take years off your appearance.

If you have any neck problems, please consult with your physician before doing any facial or neck exercises.

5)   Iolight Enhancer Kit or Facial Spoon

There are two products I have used and those products are an Iolight Machine and Facial Spoon. These machines do basically the same thing, they heat up slightly and that heat helps to penetrate your facial serums, lotions or creams into the skin. If you feel like having a spa treatment, just indulge yourself. Place a small amount of serum, lotion or cream on your face then turn on your Iolight machine or facial spoon and let the heat penetrate into your skin to temporarily reduce the appearance of fine lines. A spa experience in the comfort of your own home, what could be a better then that? We all deserve to pamper ourselves from time to time and now we can.

6)   Dermal Enhancer Tool

Another beauty enhancing device is the Dermal Enhancer Tool and this tool uses a low micro current and/or mild vibration up to 30 times pre minute and can enhance the performance of creams. By using this tool, you will see a significant improvement in the appearance of roughness, fine lines and wrinkles. The improvements can be seen in as little as one month. (All Skin Types)

(Home Shopping Network) or (beauty supplies) or (internet.)

7)   IGIÁ Therma-Cleanse, Seaweed Paraffin Wax

I have also purchased another facial treatment product and that treatment is the IGIÁ Therma-Cleanse, Seaweed Paraffin Wax. This treatment is comparable to the treatment given to your hands when you go to the spa and get a paraffin wax treatment except you put the paraffin wax on your face.

This treatment consists of a Therma-cleanse unit, brush and facial masks and the seaweed mud paraffin. Besides the seaweed mask you can order other beneficial paraffin facial wax treatments such as avocado, apricot, grade seed and more.

This machine comes with Vitamin-C Serum to help fight and repair the signs of aging. I apply the Vitamin-C Serum and then I apply three or four layers of the seaweed paraffin wax, I wait 10 minutes and remove. The penetration benefits are remarkable. The warm paraffin wax coats your face like a second layer of skin, locking in heat and moisture. It opens up the pores, allowing the age defying nutrients to penetrate deep to loosen dirt, oil and impurities.

It is imperative that you test the wax on small portion of your face before applying to the entire face and neck area. Some persons may not be able to tolerate the intense heat. I find it comfortable for my skin type. I use this machine twice a week. (All Skin Types)
(IGIA) (www.igia.com)

After you have exercised and toned your face, neck and eye muscles, you will be ready to start taking proper care of your skin.

There are steps that you should go through to take proper care of your skin. In doing so, you will reduce the fine lines and wrinkles and even out your skin tone revealing a more vibrant, glowing and youthful appearance.

The series of steps that should be followed to achieve a more youthful appearance are mentioned below:

1. Removing Makeup
2. Cleansers
3. Toners, Astringents and Clarifiers
4. Exfoliators
5. Vitamins/Serums
6. Moisturizers
7. Lifting/Firming Products/Masks

   8.   Procedures

   9.   Homemade Skin Care

If you have delicate or sensitive skin, test any new skin care product on a small inconspicuous area on your face, preferably near the ear or jawbone, to see if your skin has a negative reaction.

If you have any questions about any of the ingredients, take the product to a dermatologist or pharmacist and ask his or her opinion. Allergic reactions can happen to anyone. Generally, most people will not have a reaction unless they have extremely sensitive skin.

I found by trying a multiplicity of skin care products that I am allergic to Vitamin K. I purchased a lotion and one of the ingredients was Vitamin K and I did not think anything of it and put it on my skin, big mistake. So I will say it one more time, please test any new skin care products on an inconspicuous area before applying to you eye, neck or face.

Now you are ready to embark on a new experimental journey. The products, techniques and procedures that I recommend will give you a more youthful appearance which in turn will give you more confidence. It is a proven fact that when you look better you will feel better and that feeling will give you more confidence.

4

Scraping Off the Top Layer Removing Makeup

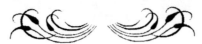

The second step in the restoration process is to remove your makeup. Most manufacturers of makeup removers will most likely advertise their product as the best product to remove makeup because of the ingredients.

When you are taking off your makeup, you do not need special additives or ingredients, you are just taking off the makeup from the surface of your skin and by doing so, you are preparing your skin for the cleansing process.

In order to remove your makeup, select a product which has a thick and creamy consistency. Removing all of your makeup before cleansing is necessary. Yes, removing your makeup and cleansing are two separate steps.

Put a small amount of make up remover on your face using warm water, never hot water, to remove your makeup. If you have sensitive skin, use your hands. If you do not have sensitive skin, use a face cloth to remove all traces of makeup.

The products which I recommend are:

1. Cold Cream, any brand (drug store)

2. Cocoa Butter, any brand (drug store)

3. Natural Herb Cleanser, any brand (Drug store)

You do not need a special makeup remover for the eye area and a special makeup remover for the face and neck areas, you just need one. Even if you have oily skin you can use a thick-creamy product because you are not leaving any of the makeup remover behind.

This step is not a science nor is it difficult but removing all of your makeup is very important. In order for a cream, lotion, gel, serum or vitamin to penetrate the skin evenly and effectively, your skin must be perfectly free of all make up.

Always keep in mind that you must never tug or pull around the delicate and sensitive eye area.

5

Away With the Grime
Cleansers

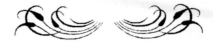

The third step in the restoration process is to cleanse your skin. Cleansing your skin is a very important step. You must remove any loose dead skin cells, excess oils, dirt, debris and free radicals that have accumulated during the course of the day. There are so many facial cleansing products on the market today; making a selection can be very confusing.

Over 40 skin does need special attention when cleansing. I have listed cleansers that perform a variety of functions. You will be able to select skin cleansers from the descriptions I have given. You will need a variety of cleansers depending on the condition of your skin on any given day. As in most cases, the condition of your skin may vary with the change of seasons and in come cases, the condition of your skin may vary each and every month.

Cleansers can be in many forms such as gels, liquids, lotions, milks and creams. You must read the labels on the cleansers the ingredients will tell you that you have made the best choice. Some cleansing products will state that their product will hydrate but it may not contain any hydrating ingredients. You must know what ingredients best fits your particular needs. You must become an informed consumer.

Look for key words, for example, glycolic or alpha hydroxy, if you find a product with either or these ingredients, that product will assist with the removal of dead skin cells. If you find a product that states that it will hydrate, look for hydrating ingredients. For example, look for words like humectants, emollients or soy because they have moisturizing properties.

After you have selected a facial cleanser, apply a small amount onto your face. With a face cloth or your hands use tepid water, washing in an upward and outward circular motion making sure to wash every inch of your skin, please include your ears and your neck, front and back. Make sure that you wash your face for approximately two to three minutes to ensure that your have completely cleansed your face, neck and eye areas, pat dry or air dry your face always remembering never to tug, pull or stretch the skin.

When cleansing, never use hot or cold water, instead, use tepid and/or cool water. Hot water dries the skin and cold water may rupture facial capillaries.

Experiment with your cleansers. You can use different cleansers during the course of the day. Depending on your skin type, select one in the morning and if need be, a different cleanser in the evening.

Just by feeling and looking at your skin you will know what cleanser your skin needs at that moment. One morning your skin may be drawn and tight and in that case, you should use a hydrating cleanser. If your skin is extra oily, use an oil free or an exfoliating cleanser.

I do use different cleansers depending on the condition of my skin that day.

The products which I recommend are:

1)   **Glycolic Cleanser**
     Serious Skin Care

     Serious Skin Care's Glycolic Cleanser 4-oz bottle is soap free and oil free. It is both extremely gentle and suitable for any skin type. This cleanser has a low pH balance for deep pore cleansing. It is formulated to help dissolve the skin build up, debris and dead skin cells.
     (All Skin Types)
     (Serious Skin Care)
     (Home Shopping Network)

2)   **Dual-Action Facial Cleanser**
     LeMirador

     Alpha Hydroxy Acid and Vitamins A, C and E, and D3. Alpha Hydroxy Acid gently opens the pores and pycnogenol (a powerful new anti-oxidant) derived from the bark of European coastal pine trees, helps prevent damage caused by free radicals. Vitamin's A, C, E, D3 and Beta-Carotene and other ingredients that will leave your skin feeling and looking soft and squeaky clean.

(All Skin Types)

(LeMirador)

(QVC) or 1800-345-1515 or (www.lemiradorskincare.com)

3) **Deep Cleanser—Cush**
    Bare Escentuals

Deep Sea Foaming Seaweed Cleanser.

This product is a blend of natural ingredients that are formulated for all skin types. The gel provides deep pore cleansing for soft, pH-balanced skin. A delicate emollient protects the skin's neutral acid mantle and helps retain moisture. Cush takes its inspiration from the sea, with a blend of nurturing sea ingredients.

(All Skin Types)

(Bare Escentuals)

(QVC) or www.Barescentuals.com

4) **Gentle Cleanser**
    Hydron

This product contains no soap or harsh detergents that will destroy your skin's natural moisturizing agents. Hydron facial cleansers for normal-to-dry and normal-to-oily skin are specifically formulated to clean your skin completely while protecting its delicate pH and moisture balance.

Cleans while hydrating, removes dirt and debris without drying your skin and is pH-balanced to protect essential oils. Conditions the skin and will prevent moisture loss from occurring.

(All Skin Types)

(Hydron Collection)

(call 1-800-4HYDRON) (www.hydron.com)

5)   **Estrosoy Facial Cleanser with Collagen**
Marilyn Miglin

Wash away dirt and oils from your face with the added benefits of nourishing emollients and collagen. Marilyn Miglin created the Estrosoy Foaming Facial Cleanser especially for women over forty to help reduce the effects of time the environment and hormonal changes. This non-drying, foamy facial cleanser contains a rich concentrated formula of three natural forms of soy to help protect the skin while washing. Skin appears softer, smoother and refreshingly cleansed. This product is great for over 40 skin.

(All Skin Types)

(Marilyn Miglin)

(Home Shopping Network)

6)   **Go Jojo: Facial Cleanser**
Sumbody

This gentle, exfoliating cleanser is full of Jojoba beads tiny scrubbing spheres in a rich creamy lotion. Excellent for sensitive or dry skin in need of an extremely gentle exfoliation. The perfect one step cleanser.

Sumbody is a line of skin care products that are handmade and fresh that contains all natural ingredients.
(All Skin Types)
(Sumbody)
(www.sumbody.com)

7) **Vita-Peptide™**
Dr. Jeannette Graf, M.D

Protein Action Cleanser
Protein-based with Vita-Peptide. This is truly skin compatible since skin is made of protein. Contains skin smoothing ingredients for gentle but effective cleansing. Gently removes dead skin cells, dirt and debris
(All Skin Types)
(Dr. Jeannette Graf)
(Home Shopping Network)

8) **Buff Polish**
Serious Skin Care

Who wants a face full of flaky, dead skin?! Yuck! Removing it will help give you fresher, younger-looking skin. Here's how: Serious Skin Care's Buff Polish acts as an exfoliating cleanser to gently buff away dead skin cells and dry flakes. Buff Polish helps give your skin a clean, polished and healthy appearance revealing a more glowing and youthful complexion.
(All Skin Types)
(Serious Skin Care)
(Home Shopping Network)

9) **Performage Cream Renewal Cleanser**
    Le Mirador

Beauty after the age of 40 begins with skin that performs at its peak. This rich, whipped Le Mirador® Performage™ cleanser transforms quickly into a cushion of foam that effortlessly lifts and floats away dirt, oil, and makeup. A creamy mixture of almond and marshmallow extract helps soothe and condition the skin, while stimulating soy, emollient avocado, and watercress soak your skin for a soft, supple, visibly bright and refreshed effect.
(All Skin Types)
(Le Mirador)
(QVC) or 1-800-345-1515
(www.lemiradorskincare.com)

10) **SilkSkin Cleanser**
    California Cosmetics

Cleanses without harsh, drying detergents, gently lifting away makeup, excess oil and microscopic dirt. Vitamin E fights free-radical damage while the homeopathic action of Calendula and Calcarea Sulphurica will condition your skin as you clean.
(All Skin Types)
(SilkSkin)
(California Cosmetics Corp.) (1-800 366-8243)

11) AHA/BHA Exfoliating Cleanser
Murad

Rich-lathering formula gently cleanses and exfoliates sur-face skin cells with a unique complex of Alpha and Beta Hydroxy Acids and Jojoba Beads. Removes surface impuri-ties, leaving skin soft, smooth and refreshed. Also contains natural hydrating agents and soothing properties. Use two to three times a week. Avoid the eye area.
(All Skin Types)
(Murad)
(1-800-336-8723) or (www.murad.com)

12) Wild Oats Scrub

Natural exfoliating cleansing scrub. Revitalizes skin's natu-ral low-deep cleaning. Contains Honey, Comfrey and Vitamin E to soften your skin. No artificial colors. When applying onto sensitive skin, add more water.
(All Skin Types)
(Wild Oats Scrub)
(Health or Natural Store)

13) Exfoliating Scrub
Principal Secret

This scrub encourages your skin's natural renewal process while lifting off dirt and pollution. It contains special man-made granules that are perfectly round and smooth to safely remove dead surface cells without causing tiny tears or irri-tation to your skin. Your face looks smoother and healthier.
(All Skin Types)

(Principle Secret
c/o Guthy Renker, Dept CTJ
P.O. Box 57054 Irvine, CA 92618-7034)
(1-800-545-5595) or (www.principalsecret.com)

14) Glucosamine Acid-Free Phyto-Pumpkin Scrub
Serious Skin Care

Say goodbye to dead, dulling facial skin with this Phyto-Pumpkin Scrub from Serious Skin Care. This special formulation is designed to gently resurface your complexion and leave the skin smooth, soft and healthy looking. The scrub helps polish and exfoliate delicate skin types without acids while added pumpkin and nut oils help condition and soften your skin.
(All Skin Types)
(Serious Skin Care)
(Home Shopping Network)

15) purity made simple facial cleanser
Philosophy

There is no reason for a second step of toning when you have a well-formulated cleanser. This easy-to-use real purity from philosophy is a four-in-one product: it is a make-up remover, a cleanser, a toner, and a light hydrator in one easy step. Purity made simple was formulated to actually emulsify and dissolve dirt, imbedded debris, and makeup rather than creating a lot of foam without a lot of clean. It is also pH balanced.
(All Skin Types)

(Philosophy)
(QVC) or (www.philosophy.com)

16) **Melting Scrub with Ginger, Honey and Pearl Powder**
Le Mirador

Melting Scrub is the future of exfoliating formulas. This advanced technology gel begins as a high-performance scrub that polishes away surface cells to reveal a younger-looking complexion. It renews tone and clarity to leave skin visibly luminous and radiant.
(Le Mirador)
(QVC) or 1-800-345-1515 (www.lemiradorskincare.com)

17) **Polished perfection Exfoliating Scrub**
Joan Rivers—Results

Joan's gentle exfoliation beads clear away all the nasty things that can dull and dirty your skin. Excess oils, make up traces, rough spots, flaking and peeling gone, gone, gone! The beads are made perfectly round and smooth, for those of us who do not want their skin irritated.
(All Skin Types)
(Joan Rivers™)
(QVC) or (www.joanrivers.com)

18) **Polishing Grains—Emerald: Facial Cleanser**
Sumbody

Facial cleanser: Let premium California rice nourish your face. It's roasted with freshwater algae from the ancient Lao capital of Luang Prabang. This is the formula to use if you are looking for anti-wrinkle cleanser.

Sumbody is a line of skin care products that are handmade and fresh that contains all natural ingredients.

(All Skin Types)

(Sumbody)

(www.sumbody.com)

19) **Gentle Deep 4-in-1 Cleanser**
Principal Secret

This is your first step toward a renewed, more youthful complexion. The Advanced Gentle Deep 4-in-1 Cleanser removes your face makeup, washes away eye makeup, cleans and tones your skin in just one simple step. Plus, it's enriched with such skin nourishing vitamins as A, B5, C and E for supple and younger-looking skin. Just apply to your moist face and rinse; you're your skin will feel soft, fresh and clean—never taut or dry.

(All Skin Types)

(Principle Secret
c/o Guthy Renker, Dept CTJ
P.O. Box 57054 Irvine, CA 92618-7034)

(1-800-545-5595) or (www.principalsecret.com)

20) **Gluosamine Acid-Free Skin Resurfacing**
Cleanser—Serious Skin Care

This product helps to remove makeup and impurities. It also assists in dissolving dull, dead skin cells. The skin feels clean, not stripped

(All Skin Types)
(Serious Skin Care)
(Home Shopping Network)

21) Olive Oil Emulsifying Cleanser—
Serious Skin Care

First Pressed Olive Oil Emulsifying Cleanser helps to dissolve dirt and makeup with maximum delivery to your skin. On contact with water, this unique cleansing oil turns into a fine, silky foam that cleans your skin without abrading the skin's soft, cushiony layer. This special formulation helps leave your skin perfectly clean and unbelievable soft without any oily residue. It has a refreshing olive oil scent and a perfect cleanser for dry and/or mature skin.
(All Skin Types)
(Serious Skin Care)
(Home Shopping Network)

22) Miraculously Younger Dry Skin Cleanser
Diane Young

Diane Young's Miraculously Younger Dry Skin Cleanser leaves skin clean and moist without that tight, dry feeling.
(Diane Young)
(QVC) or www.dianeyoung.com

Some days you will want a gentle cleanser while other days you will want an exfoliating or hydrating cleanser. Above, you have a variety of cleansing products to choose from. I use different cleansers depending on what I feel my skin needs at that particular time. All you have to do is look at and feel your skin and by doing so, you will know exactly what type of cleanser your skin will need.

Your new beauty regimen starts with clean healthy skin. I have selected the best possible skin cleansers for aging skin. All you have to do is to select a few products that will enhance your skin type.

As usual if you have sensitive skin, test any new product on an inconspicuous area before applying.

6

Tone Your Body/Tone Your Skin
Toners, Astringents and Clarifiers

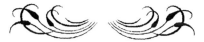

The fourth step in the restoration process, after you have cleansed is to apply a toner, clarifier or astringent. This step will complete the cleansing process. It will also, in most cases, restore the pH balance that cleansing may have depleted.

There are many types of skin toners available for women today, including: Astringents, Toners, Clarifiers and more.

There are toners, astringents that help control oil, toners that hydrate your skin and toners that will tighten the skin. You also have clarifiers that will help to even out your skin tone.

A good toner, astringent or clarifier will make your skin feel fresh, toned and in some cases, minimize the appearance of your pore size.

Some facial toners, astringents and clarifiers will rebalance your skin's fragile chemistry while others are made for T-zone, problem skin and combination or oily skin. For the most part an astringent will draw together or constrict soft tissues.

By using the appropriate product for your particular skin type, it will accelerate the removal of fine lines, and wrinkles and other signs of aging. By removing excess residue, your skin will be restored to its natural pH balance.

What exactly is pH balance? Again we have to go back to the diet. Restoring the pH balance starts with a proper nutritious diet. This will include eating alkalizing foods, low sugar fruits, vegetables and supplements, etc. You should not ingest refined sugar if at all possible. In order to rebalance your skin after using a harsh cleanser or exfoliation product, you should use a pH balance toner. By immediately restoring the skin's natural pH factor, you have restored your skin's acid mantle which covers your skin. The destruction of the pH balance in your skin will produce fine lines, wrinkles and a host of other skin issues. Healthy skin maintains a pH level between 4.5 and 5.5 Restoring the skin's pH balance will increase the skin's ability to receive nourishment from your treatment products and moisturizers.

There are also gentle products designed to hydrate and calm sensitive skin decreasing the probability of inflammation or irritation.

Using a toner, clarifier or astringent is the last opportunity you will have to remove any remaining oil, dirt, debris and residue before applying your skin care products.

The best way to choose the best product for your particular needs will be to read the label and look for the ingredients that will best complement your skin's needs.

When toning, put the product of your choice on a cotton ball applying it in an upward-circular motion. It is important to remember that you should not use a toner, astringent or clarifier around the eye area unless the product you have selected specifically says that it can be used near the eye area.

The products which I recommend are:

1) **Toner—Alcohol Free**
   Hydron

   Botanical toner—freshens, purifies and is alcohol-free. This toner gently removing the final traces of your cleanser, makeup and grime without drying skin or stripping your skin of natural humectants. Protects your skin's natural moisture balance while moisturizing it to receive maximum Hydron moisturizing benefits. Leaves your skin feeling fresh and exhilarated. Hydron is pH-balanced—oil balancing-controls shine without drying your skin.
   (All Skin Types)
   (Hydron Collection)
   (1-800-4HYDRON) or (www.hydron.com)

2)   **Clarifier—Tri-Activating Clarifier**
      # Hydron

Non-irritating blend of Alpha Beta and Poly Hydroxy Acids penetrates quickly and is oil-free. Uncovers a brighter, more radiant complexion by enhancing your skin's natural renewal process with a non-irritating blend of Alpha, Beta and Poly Hydroxy Acids. It works gradually to improve evenness of tone, skin translucency, resilience and elasticity.
(All Skin Types)
(Hydron Collection)
(or call 1-800-4HYDRON) or (www.hydron.com)

3)   **Clarifying Astringent—Alcohol-Free Formula for Oily Prone Skin**
      Murad

Witch Hazel tightens pores without drying. Calendula Extract calms irritated skin. Algae and Cucumber Extracts prevent dehydration. Lemon Extract's astringent properties balance oily skin. Cools blemished skin. Grape See and Green tea Extracts provide antioxidant protection.
(Murad)
(Oily Prone Skin)
(1-800 336-8723) or (www.murad.com)

4)   **Toner—Cush Toner**
      Bare Escentuals

Equilibrium Sea Facial Tonic from Bare Escentuals is a mild, yet effective facial toner suited for most skin types.

Use in conjunction with a cleanser to help remove traces of oil and makeup that cling to the skin even after rising. Soothing and refreshing, it contains antioxidants with the infusions of algae, kelp, witch hazel, cucumber and ivy extracts.
(Bare Escentuals)
(QVC) or (www.bareescentuals.com)

5) **SilkSkin Toner**
California Cosmetics

Is an alcohol free astringent comprised of pure distilled Witch Hazel plus Selenium for oil balance and homeopathic ingredients Thuja Occidentalis for its natural anti-bacterial action. Toner helps restore your skin's pH balance, removes trace residue and assists in minimizing pore size.
(All Skin Types)
(SilkSkin)
(California Cosmetics Corp.) (1-800-366-8243)

6) **Hydrating Toner**
Murad

Algae, Chamomile and Cucumber Extracts soothe and infuse skin with hydrating moisture. Peach Extract softens dry skin. Grape Seed Extract and Vitamins C and E provide protection from free radicals. Chamomile acts as an anti-inflammatory. It is the perfect complement to your daily skin care regimen. Murad has a toner for all skin types.
(Murad) mild
(1-800-336-8723) or (www.murad.com)

7)   **Absolutely Magic Brightening Toner**
      Results
      Joan Rivers

Do you believe in Magic? You will once you try Joan Rivers Absolutely Magic Brightening Toner. Formulated with 2% hydroquinone, this toner helps fade age spots, freckles, and hyper-pigmentation so your skin looks more radiant. (Joan River™)
(QVC) or (www.joanrivers.com)

Above I have listed numerous tones, astringents and clarifiers for you to choose. As always, knowing your skin type is very important when selecting any new products.

If you have sensitive skin, test any new product on an inconspicuous area of the face before applying.

Pores

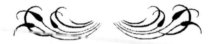

After you have taken off your makeup and cleansed your face but before you tone, give your enlarged pores the extra attention they need.

The face has over 20,000 pores and those of us with enlarged pores; should perform this extra step. A pore minimizing product will give your pores the appearance of being smaller. The sad fact is for the most part; your pore size is inherited or they can become enlarged by constant sun exposure.

After the age of 40 the increasing sun exposure you have experienced over the years will breakdown your skin's collagen level and this breakdown will manifest itself in the loss of your skin's elasticity and resilience; therefore, permanently enlarging the size of your pores. Enlarged pores also results from the over activity of the sebaceous glands which causes the pores to get clogged thus stretching the pores.

One way to minimize the appearance of your pores would be to steam your face. Once a week, steam your face before applying a pore minimizing product. When your pores are clean and free of impurities such as oil, dirt and debris and dead skin cells they appear smaller.

When you steam your face you are causing your blood vessels to dilate and by doing so, your skin will swell to some extent giving your pores the appearance of being smaller.

Steam cleaning your face will assist with lifting out the dirt, debris and the accumulation of dead skin cells. The most important task that you can perform is to keep your pores clean. The second most important step you can perform regarding your pores is to keep them clean.

It would be best for your skin if you would perform the pore minimizing step two or three times a week if possible. Please note that you must find your own comfort level. Every person is different and it is through trial and error that you will find what is right for you and your skin type.

After applying the pore minimizing product and leaving it on for the allotted time period, rinse with warm water and then splash with cool water.

As always, test any new product before using. One of the reasons pores may be more apparent is your poor exfoliation habits.

The products which I recommend are:

1) **Pore Strips**

    Using these strips will effectively pull out dirt, excess oil and debris from clogged pores giving your pores the appearance of being smaller.
    Any Brand (Drug Store)

2) **Triple Glycolic Mask Deep Pore Cleanser**
    Serious Skin Care

    Your red and irritated skin will benefit from the deep-pore cleansing action in Serious Skin Care's Triple Acting Glycolic Mask. Use it to remove oil and skin-cell debris, and then apply a light layer over face, forehead and neck. Allow to dry for 5-7 minutes. Wash off with warm water for a clean, refreshing feeling. Cleans pores of oil, dirt,

debris and dead skin cells giving your pores the appearance of being smaller.
(All Skin Types)
(Serious Skin Care)
(Home Shopping Network)

3) **Unplugged**
    Serious Skin Care

The new double strength Serious Skin Care Unplugged is a serious skin balancer, minimizing the appearance of dead surface cells and complexion dulling impurities. Daily use of Unplugged helps give skin a clearer more healthy appearance by balancing the oil content without excess drying.
(Serious Skin Care)
(Home Shopping Network)

4) **Drug Store Brand—Self-Heating Masks**

One minute deep cleansing treatment. Specifically formulated to help open and deeply cleanse pores and removes impurities. Just by adding water, the product heats on your face and will remove the pore clogging matter that has collected during the course of the day.
(Any Brand) (Drug Store)

5) **Self-Heating Mask**
    Serious Skin Care

Deep cleans the face, gets rid of debris giving you a radiant complexion. The mask works by heat, removing impurities

from the skin. The self-heating mask will leave your skin smooth, clean, refreshed and healthier-looking while diminishing the appearance of your pores.
(All Skin Types)
(Serious Skin Care)
(Home Shopping Network)

6)   **Scrub and Masque**
     Kiss My Face

Almond, Oat and Corn combined with clay and our local honey stimulates circulation, absorbs impurities, and reduces enlarged pores. Use daily as a gentle scrub, weekly as a firming and deep cleansing masque. You will see a reduction in the size of your pores.
(All Skin Types)
(Health Food Store)
(www.kissmyface.com) or (Kiss My Face, Corp.—P.O. Box 224, Gardiner, NY 12525)

7)   **Olive Oil Hydration Mask**
     Serious Skin Care

Help take care of your skin with this Olive Oil Hydration Mask from Serious Skin Care. It's infused with natural clay from the earth as well as rich, golden olive oils and olive leaf extract. The mask helps provide a deep, yet gentle pore cleansing. Use weekly as a super hydration beauty treatment and enjoy a calm, comfortable feel.
(Serious Skin Care)
(Home Shopping Network)

8)   **It's About Time Face Mask**
     Sumbody

Loaded with every natural ingredient we could find, including Vitamin C to brighten, DMAE for its time-reversing effects, and vitamins to rejuvenate and make your skin look younger, more vibrant, and incredibly youthful! One-hundred and ten percent (110%) natural ingredients bring you a face mask that is excellent for deep pore cleansing and perfect for those in need of a pore-minimizing, anti-aging, anti-oxidant miracle worker.
Sumbody is a line of skin care products that are handmade and fresh that contains all natural ingredients.
(All Skin Types)
(Sumbody) (www.sumbody.com)

9)   **Reverse HD High Definition Diffuser**
     Serious Skin Care

Look your best and youngest every day. This beauty treatment in a 1 oz. bottle is formulated with Argifirm. It helps create a unique soft focus by instantly and temporarily minimizing the look of fine lines, wrinkles and enlarged pores. SSC's Reverse HD primes the skin and creates a surface sealing effect—helping to keep important moisture in. Special light reflectors work to diffuse the look of the skin's irregularities by maintaining equal levels of light and shadow.
(Serious Skin Care)
(Home Shopping Network)

Note: For those of us with enlarged pores, after you have put on your moisturizer but before you apply your makeup, use:

A Primer with Silicone
Serious Skin Care

Give your complexion a new, smooth look with the help of Serious Skin Care's A-Primer. This oil free, Vitamin A line filler glides over your skin, filling in lines, wrinkles and pores with amazing silicones and luminous light reflectors to help create a smooth, flawless appearance. And to ease makeup application, A-Primer with retinyl palmitate allows liquid and/or powder foundation to go on evenly with remarkable ease. A-Primer helps your skin feel and look polished and luminous
(All Skin Types)
(Serious Skin Care)
(Home Shopping Network)

Lips

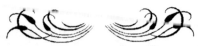

The lip area is another problem area. As we get older our lips and the area around the mouth will need special attention. One powerful antioxidant for the lip area is vitamin E. This antioxidant helps prevent the premature signs of aging, while restoring moisture to the surface of the lips.

Exfoliating accelerates cell renewal to smooth lines giving them a fuller, smoother more youthful appearance. Apply a small amount of your favorite exfoliating product onto a soft tooth brush and brush you lips thus getting rid of any accumulation of dead skin cells. If you have sensitive skin, however, just exfoliate your lips and the area around the lips with a soft tooth brush.

After exfoliating your lips with a product made especially for this area, apply one of the products that I have listed below to the lips and lip area and the results will be very gratifying within two to four weeks.

Before going to bed, protect your lips with a thin layer of Vitamin-E Oil thus locking in moisture, or any product specifically designed to moisturize the lips.

The products which I recommend are:

1) **Coneflower Lip Line Firmer**
    Diane Young

    Temporarily fills in the lines but is also a treatment. The benefits are immediate while the skin around the mouth is getting a long-term treatment. Put the lip line firmer around the lip area to prevent your lipstick from bleeding upward and downward into your fine lines. Put a little directly onto your lips before applying your lipstick, the lipstick will stay on longer. Over time, it gently exfoliates, tones and firms for a smoother, younger look.
    (All Skin Types)

(Diane Young)
(QVC) or (www.dianeyoung.com)

2) **Lip Line Anti-Feathering Treatment**
    Principal Secret

Antioxidant, anti-feathering treatment conditions your lips and helps diminish the appearance of fine lines around your lips. Dermatologist tested, and hypoallergenic. Contains Vitamins A, C, E and Grape-Seed extract to help restore your lovely, supple lips.
(All Skin Types)
(Principal Secret—c/o Guthy Renker, Dept CTJ—P.O. Box 57054—Irvine, CA 92618-7034) or(1-800-545-5595) or (www.principalsecret.com)

3) **Megalip—Directly on the lips**
    Parthena

This product will give you fuller, plumper, firmer, softer looking lips within 29 days. This product exfoliates and softens your lips giving them a fuller and softer appearance
(All Skin Types)
(Parthena)
write to: Parthena Cosmetics, LLC., 4001 S. Decatur Blvd., Suite 37-230, Las Vegas, NV 89103-6554

4) **Lip Therapy Duo**
    Le Mirador

This lip duo contains a gentle exfoliating peel and a moisture stick with Tea Tree Oil with an SPF 15 protection. The

cool refreshing peel exfoliates chapped, rough lips with gentle AHAs and brings them to silky, smooth, kissable condition. The unique two tone formula moisturizes and protects against environmental damage.
(All Skin Types)
(LeMirador)
(QVC) or 1-800-345-1515—(www.lemiradorskincare.com)

5) **Lips—Directly on the Lips**
Alpha Hydrox

Contains SPF 8 Sunscreen. Lasting lip treatment protects, heals and relieves lip drying with moisturizers enriched with Lactic healing oils, and sunscreen. ProVitamins A, E and D3, natural healing oils and sunscreen. Daily use will keep your lips looking and feeling healthy, smooth and soft giving them a fuller appearance.
(All Skin Types)
(Alpha Hydrox) www.alphahydrox.com
(Drug Store) or Neoteric Cosmetics, Inc., P.O. Box 39-S, Denver, CO 80239 or 1-800-55 ALPHA)

7

Scrubbing Off the Years
Exfoliators

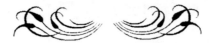

The fifth step in the restoration process is to exfoliate your skin. Exfoliating your face, neck and eye areas, I feel, is the most important part of the skin restoration process.

The removal of dead skin cells will reveal a more youthful, healthy and radiant complexion. Your fine lines and wrinkles will be diminished and the color and texture of your skin will be more even giving you a more youthful appearance. If the surface of your skin has an accumulation of dead skin cells, those cells will settle into your fine lines, wrinkles and pores giving your skin an aged appearance.

All skin types have dead skin cells that produce at an enormous rate. As we get older, it is more difficult to remove them without a product made specifically for that particular purpose.

Exfoliating products are used to remove the dead skin cells that cling to the surface of your skin. I strongly recommend, if you have more than a few fine lines and even if that is all you have, to undergo a procedure (some type of exfoliation process) in addition to purchasing exfoliating products.

I have had two peels one peel was mild while the other was much more intense. It was after my facial peel experience that I decided to have another exfoliating process and that process was called microdermabrasion. Please note that both processes will be explained in length in Chapter 9.

All three procedures will accelerate the removal of the outer-most layer of skin which will even out your skin tone, minimize your fine lines and diminish the depth of your wrinkles. The removal of those dead skin cells will allow new skin to grow and that new skin will be healthy giving you a younger appearance.

Whether you decide to undergo an exfoliating procedure or not, the number of times you exfoliate your skin will depend on your skin type and the condition of your skin. You do not want to over exfoliate your skin, by over exfoliating you will strip your face of protective oils. Please consult with a dermatologist. He or she will tell you what type of skin you have and what type of procedure is best for you and will also let you know the number of times per week you should exfoliate your skin. The products will vary in strength.

Knowing your skin type and the sensitivity of your skin are important factors before selecting any exfoliating product.

There are exfoliating products for the face, neck and eye areas. Remember when you exfoliate, you should not only exfoliate your face and eye areas but you should also exfoliate your neck area, <u>front and back</u>.

Before you put an exfoliating product near the eye area, make sure the product information states that this particular product may be used under the eye area and if you wish, you may also ask your dermatologist.

If you do not exfoliate your skin, it will not matter what type of skin care products you use because it will not be able to penetrate the skin properly and the intensity of the product will be severely diminished. If you do not exfoliate, you will just be putting new skin care products on top of discolored dead skin cells. The dead skin cells must be removed in order to achieve the best possible skin absorbing conditions.

I have found that the best time to exfoliate the skin is in the evening. After using an exfoliating product for approximately two weeks, switch to a milder or even stronger product. I use different exfoliating products so that my skin does not build up a tolerance for any one particular product.

The products which I recommend are:

1) **Lotion Plus 10% or 12%**
    Gly Derm

    This product contains glycolic acid which is esterified, a process that combines glycolic acid with fruit and fruit alcohols. The process produces gentle esters that maintain their full strength but are much less irritating to the skin. This lotion will reduce skin wrinkling, fine lines, dryness, roughness, flaking, scaling and restores elasticity.
    (Gly Derm)(strong)
    (dermatologist) or write to: ICN Plaza, 3300 Hyland Avenue, Costa Mesa, CA 92626 or 1-800-556-1937 or buy Gly Derm products on line.

2) **At Home Mini Facial Peel Program**
    Serious Skin Care

    Easy as 1...2...3! This gentle at-home mini peel is ideal for sensitive skin. Premeasured towelettes increase in strength as you peel your way through the 6-week program exfoliating dead, dry skin cells, revealing fresher, younger-looking skin. Ingredients include Vitamins A and C, Green Tea Extract and Papain Extract which scavenge those nasty free radicals and allow the skin's natural restorative process to continue. Skin appears clearer, smoother and more balanced. Kit comes with a sample towelette to test sensitivity.
    (Serious Skin Care)
    (Home Shopping Network) mild

3)   **Murad Treatment Combination Skin Formula**
     Murad

This product is for combination skin. Exfoliating gel balances normal and combination skin. Salicylic Acid controls occasional acne, Linoleic Acid (Vitamin F) creates a balance between oily and dry areas Glycolic Acid gently exfoliates and retextures surface skin Grape Seed Extract and Vitamins C and E fights free radicals. Murad has exfoliating products for all skin types.
(Murad)strong
(1-800-336-8723) or (www.murad.com)

4)   **Dermanew Microdermabrasion**
     Skin Care System-

Ideal for gentle yet, effective skin exfoliation and can be used alone or with your own skin care system. This system is a safe and effective alternative to chemical and laser peels. This system consists of a resurfacing tool, a 60-day supply of patented Dermanew Cream, 3 foam applicators, 1 massage attachment and 2AA batteries. The Dermanew Cream contains a naturally derived Corundum Crystal, a patented formula for optimum exfoliation and cellular rejuvenation which contains essential vitamins A, C and E and other antioxidants from repair, normalizing cell function and maximum benefits. The complex also moisturizes and hydrates to maintain skin's delicate moisture balance.
(All Skin Types)mild
(Dermanew) (1-866-44-DERMA or E-mail:
info@dermanew.com or QVC or (www.dermanew.com)

5) **AHA Facial Treatment Enhanced Cream**
   10% AHA
   Alpha Hydrox

   Smoothes surface imperfections caused by aging and sun damage. Safely and naturally exfoliates dead cells from the skin's surface to revitalize and help maintain youthful, healthy, radiant skin. Dramatically and rapidly improves surface texture, tone and firmness of skin. Free of oil, alcohol and fragrance. Ultra-light. Absorbs instantly. Contains Alpha Hydroxy Acid (Glycolic Acid: 10% of a pure 70% solution) (Alpha Hydrox)
   (Not for delicate/sensitive skin)
   (Drug Store) www.alphahydrox.com

6) **Anti-Oxidant Night Cream with AHA and**
   Pycnogenol®
   Le Mirador

   This luxurious night cream helps to reactivate damaged skin and helps to protect against further attack by free radicals and other collagen-damaging elements. A key ingredient is Pycnogenol, a patented European bioflavonoid with anti-oxidant capabilities many times greater than traditional anti-oxidants. It also contains Beta-carotene, Vitamin's A, C and E. Aloe Vera, etc. Additionally, this formula contains gently buffered alpha-hydroxy acids (AHA) to assist in exfoliating dead skin, promoting skin renewal and improving texture.
   (LeMirador)mild
   (QVC) or 1-800-345-1515
   (www.lemiradorskincare.com)

7)   **RETINOL NIGHT RESQ**
      Alpha Hydrox

This product contains pure-active Vitamin A (Retinol) with an effective pH 4. It is an anti-wrinkle firming complex which is fragrance free and has a timed released system. This formula also contains Vitamin C and Vitamin E (antioxidants).
(Alpha Hydrox)mild
(Not for delicate/sensitive skin)
(Drug Store) (www.alphahydrox.com)

8)   **Night Reform**
      Murad

Let Night Reform work at replenishing your skin while you sleep Phytoceramides replenish your skin lipids and increase moisture retention, while glycolic acid exfoliates and oat beta-glucan firms, moisturizes, and conditions. As a topper, biovectors with grape seed extract and liposomes and Vitamin's C and E work as antioxidant protectors leaving your skin both healthy and ready for the day ahead.
(Murad)strong
(1-800-336-8723) or (www.murad.com)

9)   **Performage AHA Soy 3 Minute Facial Peel**
      LeMirador

Beauty in a minute! Give your skin a three-minute makeover with a top-speed facial peel. Ultra-quick and easy, this Le Mirador ® Performage ™ facial peel provides you with a pampering luxury that won't take up too much of your time. Simply apply the peel pad over your skin to rejuvenate skin with 10% alpha hydroxyl acids and tomato and grape seed extracts. Three minutes later, swipe the neutralizer pad over the skin. The neutralizer pad stops the peeling process and leaves your skin nourished and protected with soy protein.

(LeMirador)strong

(QVC) or 1-800-345-1515 (www.lemiradorskincare.com)

10) Skin Perfect Microdermabrasion Cream Peel
Dr. Jeannette Graf

Give your complexion the ultimate beauty treatment in the comfort of your own home. Dr. Graf's Skin perfect Microdermabrasion Cream Peel deep cleanses to help reduce uneven skin tones and roughness. While not as dramatic as a medical procedure, it is a safe, effective and affordable cosmetic alternative to other more expensive skin renewal treatments such as chemical and laser peels typically done by dermatologists.

(Dr. Jeannette Graf)strong

(QVC)

11) Enzyme Appeal Salon Treatment Mask
Diane Young

Help smooth and retexturize the surface of your skin with this unique exfoliating mask that combines papaya in a cream base. The included angled applicator brush allows for the gentle application of the mask. This special treat can be used up to four times a month.

Diane Young)mild
(QVC) or (www.dianeyoung.com)

12) **2-piece vitamin C microdelivery peel**
Philosophy

Philosophy brings you an in-home Vitamin C microdelivery peel. Ideal for sun-damaged, pigmented skin, this soothing treatment gives your face the royal treatment. The bicarbonate Vitamin C crystals help to gently resurface the skin; remove dead and dry skin cells; and rejuvenate dull, sun-damaged complexions. Infusing the skin with vitamin C, the rapid activation gel gently removes dead skin cells as it aids in restoring sun-damaged skin.
(Philosophy)
(QVC) or (www.philosophy.com)

13) **save me p.m. retinol/vitamin c/peptide for fine-lines, wrinkles and uneven skin tone.**
Philosophy

Philosophy: cross training your skin is possible, topical retinol gives your skin a cardio workout by rapidly turning over skin cells, topical Vitamin C is like yoga for your skin, it gives your skin inner health and an outer glow. Topical peptides are like weight training for your skin, peptides help to lift and firm your skin. Wake up to a brighter you! Infused with a stable form of vitamin C to help brighten your skin tone, the innovative formula also aids in soothing fine lines and wrinkles.
(Philosophy)
(QVC) or (www.philosophy.com)

14) C-Extreme Results—2 part beauty treatment
Serious Skin Care

This at-tome skin resurfacing kit is a 2-part beauty treatment that helps rapidly exfoliate your skin while delivering
Vitamin C. This product is a must for over 40, mature
skin. C-Extreme Results helps your skin look smoother
and younger after just one beauty treatment. Skin feels
incredibly soft and silky. C-Extreme Results is fast, easy-to-
use, and the beauty results are fabulous! This C-No wrinkle
kit includes: 2 oz. C-Resurface—step 1 in your beauty
treatment. Apply a generous amount over clean, dry skin,
using gentle, tiny circular motion. Leave C-Resurface on
your skin for about three minutes 2 oz. C-Potion—step 2
in the beauty treatment. Apply C-Potion gel over the C-
Resurface and massage in a thin layer. You should feel a
warming sensation and see a white foaming action begin.
Leave on for one minute then rinse.
(Serious Skin Care)
(Home Shopping Club)

15) A-Peel Vitamin A DermApeel Set
Serious Skin Care

Now you can do a salon type DermApeel facial right in your
own home. This is a two-step program that provides the
products and tools you need to help you improve the overall clarity of your skin. This easy-to-use kit should be used
three times a week for best skin-beautifying results. This kit
contains: 2 oz A-Peel—the first step. A-Peel features

Vitamin A and other skin enhancing ingredients like alpha hydroxyl, glycolic and lactic acids, beta hydroxyl salicylic, malic and plus papaya and papain enzymes. 2 oz. A-Neutralizer—the second step. A-Neutralizer stops the exfoliation and pampers your skin with vitamins and soothing aloe vera. Mist over your skin and allow your complexion to drink in this rejuvenating comfort veil.
(Serious Skin Care)
(Home Shopping Network) mild

16) **Sensibrasion Peel and Seal Duo**
Serious Skin Care

Take the spa home with you! Serious Skin Care has created a two-step, acid-free microdermabrasion facial peel that you can perform in the privacy of your own home. Step one is the Sensibrasion Facial Peel. This acid-free formula allows even the most sensitive skin to benefit for this spa like peel. The rapid exfoliator contains natural fruit extracts and soft, rounded microbeads that help gently "peel" away dead, dulling debris to reveal a fresher, younger-looking complexion. Step two is the Sensibrasion Post Peel Seal. The seal is a surge of rich emollients and comforting skin smoothers that help hydrate and pamper your newly refreshed complexion.
(Serious Skin Care)
(Home Shopping Network) mild

17) **Apricot Scrub**

An effective Apricot Scrub gently scrubs away dull surface cells to reveal clean, fresh, healthy looking skin. The drug store has a wide variety of Apricot Scrubs to select from. An Apricot Scrub is a mild exfoliating product that is gentle enough to use every day. This product will unclog your pores, and will gently remove complexion-dulling dead skin cells to reveal a healthier and fresher appearance. (All Skin Types)—(Drug Store)

8

Vitamins In, Vitamins Out Vitamins and Serums

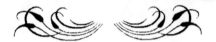

The sixth step in the restoration process is vitamins and serums. Just as our body needs vitamins from the foods we eat and/or vitamin supplements we ingest, so does our skin. Putting a vitamin supplement into our body is not enough.

The most widely used vitamins for the skin are Vitamins A, B-3, B-5, C, E and K. Applying vitamins directly onto the skin will reduce fine lines and wrinkles, tone and tighten the skin and even out the skin tone while protecting it from environmental damage. Some vitamins will assist with skin exfoliation while others will assist with skin firming and/or hydration, etc.

You will be able to determine which vitamins your particular skin type needs by the descriptions below.

The most widely used vitamins are:

Vitamin A—works as an antioxidant on the skin, meaning that Vitamin A disarms free-radical molecules. A derivative of Vitamin A; namely, Retinoic Acid is an ingredient in Retin-A and Renova, which can fade brown spots, reduce wrinkles and smooth the surface of the skin. When purchasing a Vitamin A product for the skin, look for Retinyl Palmitate, Retinyl Acetate, Retinol or Retinyl Linoleate.

Vitamin's B-3 (Niacin) and B-5 (Pantothenic Acid)—these vitamins help hold in moisture. If your skin is hydrated it is less likely to become irritated. If your skin is well hydrated your fine lines and wrinkles are diminished because your skin will attract moisture from the air and in turn, your skin will be plump and moist.

Vitamin C—is an antioxidant working to neutralize the damaging free radical molecules in the skin. Vitamin C also helps to protect your skin from the harmful effects of the sun's UVA and UVB rays which can lead to skin damage. A new vitamin in the cosmetic industry is **Vitamin C-Ester (Ascorbyl Palmitate)**. This vitamin may actually reverse existing sun damage and can be found in many non-prescription moisturizers.

Vitamin E—is an antioxidant that when added to a sunscreen, may provide additional protection from the UVB rays of the sun. This vitamin has great moisturizing properties.

Vitamin D—Vitamin D stimulates cell growth and deeply moisturizes malnourished skin. Vitamin D added to skin care products, provides healthier looking skin to those with mal-nourished, dry, irritated, and shallow skin. It will deeply mois-turize while stimulating cell growth and nourish delicate skin.

Vitamin K—will diminish broken facial capillaries and spi-der veins giving you a more flawless appearance.

The products which I recommend are:

1) **A-Force Serum with Retinol**
    Serious Skin Care

    Your skin may be starting to age, but it doesn't have to look that way. Serious Skin Care brings you the 1 oz. A-Force Serum from the A-Defiance line of skin care products. This oil-free serum is designed to help reduce the appearance of fine lines and wrinkles. The serum contains powerful antioxidants to help improve skin's texture and appearance. A-Force is clinically tested to be non-irritating and is der-matologist tested.
    (Serious Skin Care)
    (Home Shopping Network)

2) **Cellular Serum**
    Murad

    Ceramides improve moisture retention. Ivy, Cucumber and Mallow Extracts moisturize and firm, Ginseng Extract improves elasticity. Chamomile and Green Tea calm while humectants bind water to the skin for maximum hydration. Great for oily skin or as a moisture booster for dry skin.

(All Skin Types)
(Murad) (1-800-336-8723) or (www.murad.com)

3) **Perfect C Firming Crème**
    Marilyn Miglin

You deserve to use quality products in your skin care regimen. Marilyn Miglin's Perfect C Firming Crème can help you achieve the youthful appearance of healthy-looking skin you desire. This terrific formulation helps guard against the risk of environmental damage with ingredients like antioxidant Vitamin C, emollients and moisture carriers. And you will find the light citrus scent of this crème irresistible. Watch fine lines and wrinkles appear smoother as your skin takes on a softer look.
(All Skin Types)
(Marilyn Miglin)
(Home Shopping Network)

4) **Vitamin-E Oil**

Pure Vitamin E Oil
Heat small amount, apply to face and neck areas before going to bed. For an extra added treat, put some on your lips. Hydrates and exfoliates
(Drug Store—Any Brand)

5) **Vitamin-A-Capsules**

Assists with skin exfoliation, reduces fine lines and wrinkles
(Drug Store)

6)   **Phytogen Lifeline to Youth Intense Treatment Serum**
     Marilyn Miglin

This formula utilizes a new patented process to extract the phytoestrogen from the flowers of clover. The double action serum by day helps hydrate firm, protect and tone your skin. By night the serum helps rejuvenate and improve the appearance of wrinkles, fine lines and thinning, aged skin. Phytogen Intense Serum helps bring a youthful-looking fresh glow to your complexion.
(All Skin Types)
(Marilyn Miglin)
(Home Shopping Network)

7)   **C-Serum Skin Conditioner**
     Serious Skin Care

Bathe your face in Serious Skin Care's Vitamin C-infused skin conditioner. C-Serum, formulated with colloidosomes, antioxidants and botanicals, aids in lessening the appearance of fine lines and wrinkles. This distinct formula helps moisturize your skin as it helps reduce the look of wrinkles.
(All Skin Types)
(Serious Skin Care)
(Home Shopping Network)

8)   **hope and a prayer**
     Philosophy

Topical Vitamin C is a powerful topical antioxidant to help protect against photo-damage. May help to even skin tone

and reduce fine lines. This product is a powder and a liquid, just mix the two together. The Vitamin C does not lose its strength because it does not become a liquid until you mix the ingredients together just before applying the mixture onto your skin. This product also contains added benefits of zinc pca, copper pca and arginine and 99.9% I-ascorbic acid.
(Philosophy)
(QVC) or (www.philosophy.com)

9) **Ester-C Serum**
    Kiss My Face

Ester-C Serum—Contains antioxidants from the patented Vitamin Ester-C plus Green Tea and essential citrus aromatics penetrate, protect and help rebuild damaged skin.
(All Skin Types)
(Kiss My Face) (Health Food Store)
(www.kissmyface.com) or (Kiss My Face, Corp.—P.O. Box 224, Gardiner, NY 12525)

10) **Anti-aging treatment with 15% Vitamin C**
    Murad

Increases skin elasticity by 42%. Pure Vitamin C encourages collagen production. Murad's patented Exclusive Renewal Complex repairs environmental damage, retards skin aging and improves skin tone. Orange, Basil and Grapefruit extracts keep skin soothed and protected.
(All Skin Types)
(Murad) (1800-336-8723) or (www.murad.com)

11) **C-No Wrinkle Face Serum**
Serious Skin Care

Help fight the look of unsightly wrinkles with this amazing C-No Wrinkle Face Conditioning Serum (1-oz.) from Serious Skin Care. The advanced Colloidosome Vitamin C formulation helps reduce the look of wrinkles. This product is rich in antioxidants and botanicals to moisturize soothe and help reduce the appearance of fine lines. Smooth gently on the face in the mornings and the evenings.
(All Skin Types)
(Serious Skin Care)
(Home Shopping Network)

12) **Reverse Lift Serum with Argifirm**
Serious Skin Care

Always look your best and youngest every day with the help of Serious Skin Care's Reverse Lift Firming Facial Serum. This easy-to-use beauty treatment in a 1 oz. bottle is formulated with our high performance, exclusive Argifirm complex. It helps smooth over fine lines, helps with the appearance of large pores and wrinkles, and helps the skin look firmer and the pores look tighter. It also helps to visually even out the skin's tone and surface, special optical light diffusers beautifying and magical effects.
(All Skin Types)
(Serious Skin Care)
(Home Shopping Network)

13) **Glucosamine-Acid-Free Resurfacing Serum**
Serious Skin Care

Take back control of your skin with this amazing Glucosamine Acid-Free Resurfacing Serum from Serious Skin Care. This product reveals the natural radiance of the skin without the force of irritating acids. The sight of fine lines, wrinkles and pores are visibly reduced. It even helps to minimize the appearance of uneven skin tones. Use in the morning and the evening and apply to the face and throat.
(All Skin Types)
(Serious Skin Care)
(Home Shopping Network)

14) **CUSH Time Peeling Serum**
Bare Escentuals

This "Life Source" Time Peeling Serum makes it possible to see younger looking skin day after day, as glycolic, latic and fruit acid allow newer healthier skin cells to surface. Also contains essential oils of Lavender, peppermint and Sage. Use the time peeling serum nightly before moisturizing.
(Bare Escentuals—CUSH)
(QVC)

15) **Perfect C Firming Cream**
Marilyn Miglin

This cream helps guard against the risk of environmental damage with ingredients like anti-oxidant Vitamin C and moisture carriers, emollients and firmers that help revitalize

the skin's appearance leaving it looking soft and toned. Watch fine lines and wrinkles appear smoother as your skin takes on a softer look.
(All Skin Types)
(Marilyn Miglin)
(Home Shopping Network)

16) **Firming Complex Serum**
LeMirador

If you face and throat are losing their youthful resilience, this two-phase serum is for you. The oil and water-based complex helps tighten and firm and keeps skin moist and supple. This serum delivers instant results and long-term benefits for visible firmer, uplifted skin.
(All Skin Types)
(LeMirador)
(QVC) or 1-800-345-1515 (www.lemiradorskincare.com)

17) **Advanced Continuous Lift Serum**
Principal Secret

The Advanced Continuous Lift contains vitamins A, C, and E, wheat proteins, marine collagen, and amino acids. These ingredients aid in rejuvenating damaged skin and enhance the overall tone and texture of the skin. Its unique ingredient complex visibly firms face, neck, and eye areas. Hypoallergenic and dermatologist tested.
(All Skin Types)
(Principle Secret
c/o Guthy Renker, Dept CTJ

P.O. Box 57054 Irvine, CA 92618-7034)
(1-800-545-5595) or (www.principalsecret.com)

18) Perfecting Serum
Murad

Silky gel locks in moisture and smoothes line lines for all skin types. Avocado Oil and Evening Primrose Oil mimic the lipids of youthful skin to smooth fine lines. Squalane, derived from olives, imparts a silky feel. Vitamin's A & E protects and smooth skin texture. This product will lock in hydration.
(All Skin Types)
(Murad)(1-800-336-8723) or (www.murad.com)

19) Anti-Aging Ampules Set
Dr. Jeannette Graf's

This Anti-Aging Ampules set was designed to help return softness and tone to your skin and give it a more youthful appearance. You receive 30 ampules that are 0.03 oz. each. This 30-day regimen consists of three phases. During the first 10 days you apply Ampule #1, for the next ten days you apply Ampule #2 and for the last ten days you apply Ampule #3. Simply rub the contents of an ampule onto your clean face and neck with your fingertips. Phase 1 will start with your skin's most external layer and helps stimulate dry and tired skin. It also helps improve elasticity of the skin. Phase 2 uses a combination of ingredients to help provide a smooth, soft look and feel. It helps rejuvenate your skin while replenishing the moisture level. Phase 3

continues to help hydrate the skin while toning for opti-mized skin elasticity. After this 30-day program you should see the visible signs of softer, more toned skin that is more youthful-looking.
(All Skin Types)
(Dr. Jeannette Graf)
(Home Shopping Network)

20) **Principal Secret Oil-Free Hydrator**
Principal Secret

The Principal Secret Oil-Control Hydrator is like a drink of water for your face. It is specially formulated to control oil, while leaving your skin feeling smoother and softer. Its exclusive vitamin bouquet contains A, C, and E to protect skin against free radicals and pollution. The SPF of 8 also protects skin from sun's damaging rays.
(All Skin Types)
(Principle Secret
c/o Guthy Renker, Dept CTJ
P.O. Box 57054 Irvine, CA 92618-7034)
(1-800-545-5595) or (www.principalsecret.com)

21) **Multi Action Lifting Treatment**
Natural Advantage

Get in touch with your youthful side. The Natural Advantage Multi-Action Lifting Treatment is an intensive lifting serum which helps smooth the appearance of fine lines and wrinkles for radiant, younger-looking skin. Using the powerful synergy of hyalauronic acid and BH complex,

the versatile cream tones and revitalizes the skin. It is also rich with active cooper and minerals such as potassium, magnesium, zinc, and vitamins B, C, and F for gorgeous, younger-looking skin.
(Natural Advantage)
(QVC)mild)
or (1800-276-7102) or (www.naturaladvantage.com)

22) **Line Smoothing Complex**
Hydron

Line Smoothing Complex incorporates a proprietary new technology that reduces the appearance of fine facial lines, and has both immediate and long-term benefits. It combines the firming and tightening qualities of certain vegetable proteins and amino acids, and the collagen and elastin enhancing attributes of a strain of red marine algae, with the moisture-holding properties of Hydron, a hydrogel or water-attracting polymer. Clinical tests by an independent laboratory showed that, used nightly; this product produced lasting results within eight weeks, including a 30% reduction in the appearance of fine facial lines, a 35% increase in hydration, a 21% increase in skin firmness, and progressive improvement in skin's resilience and elasticity.
(All Skin Types)
(Hydron Collection)
(or call 1-800-4HYDRON) for more information or call 1-800-944-9999 to place an order or (www.hydron.com)

23) You'll C It: Facial Serum
Sumbody

Vitamin C in a form your skin can actually absorb. The benefits of Vitamin C on your skin are legendary and its benefits legion. Very few serums on the market today, however, have Vitamin C in a form your skin can actually absorb. Ours is both oil and water soluble resulting in deeper penetration of the vitamins (and results.) Packed full of natural anti-oxidants, free radical fighters and enzymes to smooth and feed your skin. This is one serum that is different than the rest. How do we know? You'll C it! Sumbody is a line of skin care products that are handmade and fresh that contains all natural ingredients.
(All Skin Types)
(Sumbody) (www.sumbody.com)

24) Miraculously Younger Skin Serum
Diane Young

A miracle in a bottle This Diane Young Miraculously Younger Anti-Aging Skin Serum combines botanicals with clinically-proven techniques to deliver anti-aging benefits. It helps reduce the appearance of fine lines and wrinkles, improve your skin's texture, and provide intense hydration. The advanced serum is excellent for all skin types.
(All Skin Types)
(Diane Young)
(QVC) or (www.dianeyoung.com)

25) **Glyco-Youth Serum**
Serious Skin Care

This serum glides on cool and smooth, veiling your face and neck with time-released Glycolic Acid. The Gentle and sustained exfoliation continues to smooth and even out your complexion in a gradual, effective manner. The serum leaves your skin feeling smooth and your complexion looking youthful, fresh and vibrant. Fine lines and wrinkles also become less noticeable.
(All Skin Types)
(Serious Skin Care)
(Home Shopping Network)

26) **Advanced Moisture with Hydrospheres**
Principal Secret

Principal Secret Advanced Moisture with Hydrospheres infuses your skin while softening fine lines, wrinkles, and other signs of aging. The patented hydrosphere delivery system contains powerful antioxidants vitamins A, C, and E. Your skin's texture, and provide intense hydration. The advanced serum is excellent for all skin types.
(All Skin Types)
(Principle Secret
c/o Guthy Renker, Dept CTJ
P.O. Box 57054 Irvine, CA 92618-7034)
(1-800-545-5595) or (www.principalsecret.com)

9

Invisible Protective Barrier Moisturizers

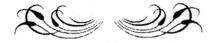

The seventh step in the restoration process is to moisturize. The main purpose of a moisturizer is to moisturize your skin while protecting it from the elements. Whether you use a moisturizer under your makeup or you decide just to put on a moisturizer and some lip gloss and go, your face must have protection. Without a protective barrier your skin will show the signs of aging at a more rapid rate because of its exposure to the elements.

Over the age of 40, you may want a moisturizer that contains beneficial restorative age-defying ingredients. Some moisturizers hydrate, some exfoliate and others may contain vitamins which are essential to the skin. There are some products today that perform multiple functions.

Protecting your skin from further damage is necessary. The sun, wind and pollution are the skin's worst enemies. There is a major repair cost if you want to reverse the damage that the elements have caused over the years. The best defense against the natural aging process is a good offense which would be a protective moisturizer. Protect your skin the best way you can. Moisturize your skin during the day and evening with anti-aging skin care products.

Moisturizers are very beneficial to your skin. Whether the moisturizer has ingredients such as Vitamin C, Vitamin A or ingredients such as humectants that attract moisture to the skin's surface you need a moisturizer.

Humectants prevent water loss from the skin by attracting moisture. If you are athletic or if you like to work in the garden or whatever outdoor activities you may participate in, you will need a sunscreen with an SPF of 30 or better. It is very important to protect your skin from the wind, sun and air pollution, etc.

If you work in an office environment or if you work at home or from home, you will most probably have the heat or air conditioner on which can also damage the skin. You must protect your skin with a moisturizer no matter what skin type you have.

If you experience minimal contact with the elements, most likely you will only require a SPF of 15, but in any case, your skin will need protection.

Some moisturizers will reverse the signs of aging while other moisturizers will protest your skin from further damage. If you are over 40, you will at some point get fine lines and wrinkles but a good moisturizer and/or sunscreen will slow the signs of aging, at least the outward aging process. It is important to know your skin type in order to effectively protect your skin from the environment.

The products which I recommend are:

1) **Reverse Lift with Argifirm Cream**
   Serious Skin Care

   Looking for an instant lift? Serious Skin Care's new and improved Reverse Lift with Argifirm may be able to help. This very special 2 oz. firming facial cream helps tighten, lift and hydrate your skin for a firmer-looking complexion with increased moisture and improved elasticity. You will love how regular use of this beauty treatment helps give you a younger look. Simply massage a generous amount of Reverse Lift gently into your face and under the jawline, using light, upward motions.
   (All Skin Types)
   (Serious Skin Care)
   (Home Shopping Network)

2) **First Pressed Olive Oil Moisture Cream**
   for the Face and Neck
   Serious Skin Care

   Pamper your dry, stressed skin with First Pressed Olive Oil Moisture Cream from Serious Skin Care. This rich cream formulated for the face and neck helps moisturize your skin with first pressed, virgin olive oil and other skin-pampering ingre-

dients. The creamy texture glides over your skin, helping to give your complexion a soft, hydrated and glowing look.
(All Skin Types)
(Serious Skin Care)
(Home Shopping Network)

3) **Hydron Line of Skin Care**
   Hydron

Hydron collections feature a variety of products essential to healthy skin and hair. A complete line of products that will hydrate the skin, reduce the appearance of fine lines and wrinkles on your face, neck and eyes. The Hydron line also consists of body and hair products for a complete youthful appearance.
(All Skin Types)
(Hydron Collection)
(or call 1-800-4HYDRON) for more information or call 1-800-944-9999 to place an order or (www.hydron.com)

4) **Skin Perfecting Lotion**
   Murad

Retexturizing, oil-free moisturizer. Honey and Meadowsweet Extracts renew skin. Retinol encourages healthy cell turnover reducing clogged pores. Algae Extract leaves skin soft and supple. Amica Extract reduces redness. Ultra light lotion leaves skin perfectly hydrated without an oily residue. Softens, revitalizes, firms and protects with lipid moisturizing systems, Retinol, antioxidants and natural conditioning agents leaves skin perfectly hydrated all day.

(All Skin Types)
(Murad) (1-800-336-8723) or (www.murad.com)

5)   **hope in a jar for dry sensitive skin**
     Philosophy

Philosophy's hope in a jar therapeutic moisturize for dry, sensitive skin is a high performance moisturizer with antioxidants to help reduce environmental damage. Our formula contains highly effective water binding agents to help preserve the skin's water/oil balance. Contains retinol and Vitamins A & E. this product is made for all skin types but specifically made for dry/sensitive skin.
(All Skin Types)
(Philosophy)
(QVC) or (www.philosophy.com)

6)   **Moisturizing Emollient**
     SilkSkin

This product contains 28 active ingredients that work synergistically to help your skin recapture its youthful qualities: skin soothing Aloe, Silk Amino Acids and Collagen to help restore firmness, along with Chamomile and other botanical nutrients. Glucose Glutamate helps lock moisture in for hours, long after most moisturizers have evaporated! My light, non-greasy Moisturizing Emollient restores and maintains smooth, supple skin without a drop of mineral oil!
(All Skin Types)
(SilkSkin)
(California Cosmetics Corp.) (1-800-366-8243)

7) **Murad Moisturizers**
    Murad

Murad has a moisturizer for All Skin Types. It does not matter what skin type you have. If you have Normal/Combination, Dry, Sensitive, Environmentally Stressed, Oily or Acne Prone Skin, Murad has a moisturizer for you. (All Skin Types)
(Murad) (1 800-336-8723) or (www.murad.com)

8) **Olay—Moisturizer**
    Olay

This is a moisturizing lotion with complete UV protection. Zinc Oxide combined with SPF 15 helps provide your skin with protection against environmental damage and the damaging UVA and UVB rays of the sun. Olay has an SPF 15 to help protect, more moisture to help prevent dryness, plus anti-oxidant vitamins E and C. It's called Complete because it is.
(All Skin Types)
(Olay)
(Drug Store) or (www.olay.com)

9) **hope in a jar—Daily Moisturizer**
    Philosophy

hope in a jar is an extra-light antioxidant moisturizing formula that may help to reduce the appearance of wrinkles and the effects of environmental damage. Also contains beta-glucan, a powerful antioxidant, which enhances skin immunology, and lactic acid, which gently exfoliates skin

to reveal smoother, healthier looking skin, for years, plastic surgeons have been recommending this formula to patients in pursuit of younger, healthier skin, results can be seen and felt within days, leaving a healthy, rosy glow to the skin that does not require makeup or cover up.
(All Skin Types)
(Philosophy)
(QVC) or (www.philosophy.com)

10) Vita Peptide—Day Moisturizer
Dr. Jeannette Graf

Natural liquid crystals penetrate the surface of the skin for enhanced release of moisture into the skin. The result: instant smoothness and softness. Vita-Peptide formula provides all-day moisture protection.
(All Skin Types)
(Dr. Jeannette Graf)
(Home Shopping Network)

11) Vita Peptide— Overnight
Dr. Jeannette Graf

Enhances and reinforces the vitality of the skin by infusing Vita-Peptide with our fortified nighttime moisture delivery complex. This unique combination replenishes the necessary ingredients for your skin to be moister, firmer and glowing. Delivers optimal moisturization during skin's nighttime renewal process and helps enhance skin's natural moisture balance.
(All Skin Types)

(Dr. Jeannette Graf)
(Home Shopping Network)

12) **Skin-Deep Wrinkle Treatment Gel**
Dr. Jeannette Graf

Helps to reverse the appearance of dry, thinning skin. This cool gel works to decrease the appearance of free-radical damage to the skin, while helping to reduce the look of medium and deep wrinkles. It will also assist in moisturizing dry, thinning skin. In just a few weeks you will see a noticeable difference.
(All Skin Types)
(Dr. Jeannette Graf—Dermatologic Formula)
(Home Shopping Network)

13) **Perfecting Night Cream**
Murad

This ultra-rich formula is designed to repair daily environmental damage, restore moisture and revitalize the skin while you sleep. The exclusive Alpha and Beta Hydroxy Acid complex improves the appearance of skin while superior antioxidants, Grape Seed Extract, Green Tea Extract and Vitamins C and E, protest against free-radical damage.
(Normal or Dry Skin)
(Murad) (1-800-336-8723) or (www.murad.com)

14) **C-No Wrinkles Moisturizer with SPF 15**
Serious Skin Care

Too much sun can definitely spoil your fun. Give your skin some much-needed protection with the Serious Skin Care C-No Wrinkle Moisturizer with SPF 15. This creamy moisturizer provides moderate protection against sunburn. Formulated with Vitamins C, A and E.
(All Skin Types)
(Serious Skin Care)
(Home Shopping Network)

15) **Hypo Allergenic Milk Plus—Skin Renewing**
Night Cream
Almay

Significantly improves the appearance of fine lines and wrinkles. Improves skin's smoothness by 48%. Renews skin clarity and radiance by 31%. Gently exfoliates and retexturizes your skin. Contains antioxidants, Vitamins A, C and E, milk protein complex fortified with Calcium. Helps to neutralize skin damaging free radicals.
(All Skin Types)
(Almay) (Drug Store)

16) **Aveeno—Skin Brightening**
Daily Moisturizer with SPF 15
Johnson and Johnson

This light, weight, fast-absorbing moisturizer contains a unique combination of naturally active complexion correctors that soften and smooth skin texture while improving

skin clarity and visibly brightening the appearance of dull-looking skin. Contains a UVA/UVB sunscreen with naturally active Soy Extract and Vitamins A and C
(All Skin Types)
(Johnson and Johnson) (1-877-298-2525) or (Drug Store)

17) **AHA Facial Treatment Enhanced Crème**
10% AHA
Alpha Hydrox

Smoothes surface imperfections caused by aging and sun damage. Safely and naturally exfoliates dead cells from the skin's surface to revitalize and help maintain youthful, healthy, radiant skin. Dramatically and rapidly improves surface texture, tone and firmness of skin. Free of oil, alcohol and fragrance. This skin care product is ultra-light and absorbs instantly. Contains Alpha Hydroxy Acid (Glycolic Acid: 10% of a pure 70% solution)
(Alpha Hydrox)
(Not for delicate/sensitive skin)
(Drug Store) (www.alphahydrox.com)

18) **Serious E Moisturizer**
Serious Skin Care

Got dry, parched skin? We have a solution! Drench it with intensive moisture and help alleviate that aging look. Serious Skin Care's Serious E Moisturizer is enriched with Vitamin E, a super antioxidant, and helps protect your skin from antioxidant damage caused by free radicals in the

environment. This thick, white moisturizer goes on freely without leaving an oily residue.
(Especially for Dry or Super Dry Skin)
(Serious Skin Care)
(Home Shopping Network)

19) A-Cream with Retinol & SPF-15
Serious Skin Care

You can use this versatile cream from Serious Skin Care every day to help reduce the look of fine lines and wrinkles. It's formulated with two million international units of Vitamin A—a powerful free radical fighter. And as an added benefit, A-Cream with Retinol and SPF-15 contains active sunscreens to help provide your delicate facial, neck or body skin with moderate protection from the sun. A-Cream is a rich, yet readily absorbed cream made to wear alone or under makeup.
(Serious Skin Care)
(Home Shopping Network)

20) Fade Cream for the Face, Hands & Body
Alpha Hydrox

Hydroquinone, plus unique ingredients from the Orient provide accelerated, superior results. Fades skin discoloration on hands, face and body caused by sun exposure, freckles, blemishes, age, pregnancy, oral contraceptives. Vitamin E and creamy emollients soften and soothe.
(Alpha Hydrox)
(Not for delicate/sensitive Skin)
(Drug Store) or (www.alphahydrox.com)

21) Triple-Action Revitalizing
    LeMirador

The winning daytime lotion keeps skin feeling soft and smooth, helps reduce the appearance of fine lines and wrinkles, and provides superior protection against premature aging for all skin types. This product contains avobenzone, which has proven to be much more effective shield from the harmful UVA rays. This facial lotion absorbs quickly and disappears into the skin to intensively hydrate and promote elasticity.
(All Skin Types)
(Le Mirador)
(QVC) or 1-800-345-1515 (www.lemiradorskincare.com)

22) **Booster Complex Renews Cell Growth**
    Principal Secret

Principal Secret's Booster Complex is a highly concentrated formula which contains a unique blend of fruit and glycolic acids that help reduce the appearance of fine lines and wrinkles while also encouraging new cell growth. Because of the presence of Vitamin E. skin tone appears more even.
(All Skin Types)
(Principle Secret
c/o Guthy Renker, Dept CTJ
P.O. Box 57054 Irvine, CA 92618-7034)
(1-800-545-5595) or (www.principalsecret.com)

23) **Facial Moisturizer—Hydrating**
Hydron

Hydron Facial Moisturizer is 100% oil-free facial moisturizer which contains humectants that hold in moisture. It has nine lipids that help strengthen the skin's natural barrier against moisture loss. It also contains antioxidant vitamins and enzymes that neutralize free radicals. SPF 15 protection, plus Avobenzone also protection you from the UVA and UVB rays of the sun.
(All Skin Types)
(Hydron Collection)
(call 1-800-4HYDRON) or (www.hydron.com)

24) **Moisture Balance Restorative**
Hydron

This product is for mature and environmentally stressed skin that needs extra moisturizing attention. Moisture Balance Restorative strengthens cells' defenses as you sleep. This ultra-rich liposome complex replenishes moisturizing agents found in healthy skin, using naturally occurring amino acids, vitamins A and E, sodium hyaluronate and vegetable lipids to improve your skin's softness and elasticity.
(Hydron Collection)
or(1-800-4HYDRON) for more information or call
1-800-944-9999 to place an order or (www.hydron.com)

25) A Good Night Cream
Serious Skin Care

Have a good night every night with Serious Skin Care! This A-good night cream is enhanced with Beta Carotene to help replenish dry skin. The lightly scented cream can help benefit aging skin by conditioning and revitalizing its texture. It also helps your skin recover from the stresses of the day so it looks younger and more vibrant in the morning. Apply cream liberally to face and neck each night for best results.
(Serious Skin Care)mild
(Home Shopping Network)

26) C-Repair Moisturizing Night Cream
Serious Skin Care

Get serious about your skin care needs with this Serious Skin Care C-Repair Moisturizing Night Cream. This luxurious night cream helps minimize the appearance of fines and wrinkles, while helping to moisturize your skin. It is designed for dry skin, comes lightly scented and goes on lightly without leaving a heavy feel. This cream is designed to help your skin look rejuvenated and revitalized.
(All Skin Types)
(Serious Skin Care)
(Home Shopping Network)

10

Lifting Up the Years
Lifting and Firming

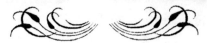

The eighth step in the restoration process is to lift and firm the skin from the neck up.

At the age of 42, I did notice a change in my skin but I was not sure exactly what that change was and I was too busy to do anything about starting a new skin care routine, well that was a big mistake on my part.

At the age of 50, I noticed that my skin tone had changed and that my skin had started to droop and sag. That is when I began to fight back. I needed to know exactly what was going on and what I could do about this change and so can you. If you are willing to be persistent and consistent you can look five, ten even fifteen years younger.

Certain products are specifically made to slightly lift the sagging skin on the face, neck and eye areas. These products come in many forms and whether the product you choose is a serum, gel, lotion or cream or a combination, they should become part of your daily skin care routine.

Some of these products will give you a slight temporary lift; I feel that they are best worn without makeup. Some work over a period of time and these products are treatments. These treatment products contain special ingredients that will slightly lift and firm the skin after a period of four to eight weeks; you should be able to actually see a difference.

There are skin care products that will restore some of the elasticity and collagen that time has depleted giving you a more firm and toned appearance. You will not find a face lift in a jar but there are products on the market today that, if used properly, can make a difference in the way you look.

If you want dramatic results, you will need cosmetic surgery but for a delicate change without surgery, select products that will give you a slightly lifted appearance.

Products which I recommend are:

1) **Facial Serum—Firms & Tightens**
   Results
   Joan Rivers

   Face boost lifting serum. This serum is a treatment that tones, tightens, firms and hydrates the skin
   (All Skin Types)

(Joan Rivers™)
(QVC) or (www.joanrivers.com)

2)   **Reverse Lift with Argifirm**
     Serious Skin Care

Looking for an instant life? Serious Skin Care's new and improved Reverse Lift with Argifirm may be able to help. This very special 2 oz. firming facial cream helps tighten, lift and hydrate your skin for a firmer-looking complexion with increased moisture and improved elasticity. You will love how with regular use of this beauty treatment it will give you a younger look. Simply massage a generous amount of Reverse Lift gently into your face and under the jawline, using light, upward motions will make a difference in the firmness of your skin.
(All Skin Types)
(Serious Skin Care)
(Home Shopping Network)

3)   **Night Reform**
     Murad

This product absorbs into skin and firms and tones while you sleep. Night Reform increases firmness by 35% so your skin feels smoother and healthier. In approximately four weeks you will see 34% fewer lines and wrinkles and an 18% increase in elasticity. Hydration is improved, skin tone is more even.
(All Skin Types)
(Murad) (1-800-336-8723) or (www.murad.com)

4) **Reverse Lift Serum with Argifirm**
Serious Skin Care

Look your best and youngest every day with the help of **Serious Skin Care's Reverse Lift Firming Facial Serum.** This easy-to-use beauty treatment in a 1 oz. bottle is formulated with our high performance, exclusive Argifirm complex. It helps smooth over fine lines, helps with the appearance of large pores and wrinkles, and helps the skin look firmer and the pores look tighter. And, to help visually even out the skin's tone and surface, special optical light diffusers act like missions of tiny micro mirrors for a beautifying and magical effect.
(All Skin Types)
(Serious Skin Care)
(Home Shopping Network)

5) **Miracle Formula Cream**
Sellecca Solution

Connie's Miracle Formula is based on ancient Egyptian beauty remedy that helps to restore skin's youthful appearance. It works to help refine skin tone and texture, improve firmness and elasticity, and visibly reduce the appearance of fine lines. Perfect for even the most sensitive skin. This dramatically different moisturizing treatment contains the rare and exotic ingredients of Frankincense, Sandalwood and Myrrh—combined with a "unique strain" of Red Marine Algae which encourages cell renewal without the irritation of harsh chemicals, dyes or perfumes and without the side

effects often associated with alpha hydroxyl acids and retinols. This miraculous super strain of Hawaiian algae naturally removes the best up, dull and dead surface cells of the skin, helping to eliminate those sticky cells that block the surface of the pores. A gently yet effective solution for sensitive skin. This unique formula works to help refine skin tone and texture, improve firmness and elasticity, and visibly reduce the appearance of fine lines.
(All Skin Types)
(Sellecca Solution) (Connie Sellecca)
(www.selleccasolution.com) or (1800-655-4333)

6)   **Advance—Continuous Lift—Serum**
Principal Secret

This product contains a unique complex of vitamins which safely lift and tighten the skin around the eyes, face and neck, and aid in rejuvenating the skin and enhancing the overall tone and appearance of the skin. Reduces the appearance of under eye bags and gives your skin a silky smooth appearance.
(All Skin Types)
(Principle Secret
c/o Guthy Renker, Dept CTJ
P.O. Box 57054 Irvine, CA 92618-7034)
(1-800-545-5595) or (www.principalsecret.com)

7)   **Years Younger Serum**
Diane Young

You will discover a more beautiful you with Diane Young's Years Younger Serum.

Contains isoflavones derived from Soy, Marine Algaes, and Concflower. This serum helps diminish the appearance of aging skin by increasing firmness. It will also decrease the appearance of fine lines and superficial wrinkles. It helps to increase skin firmness and boost skin hydration. Helps to diminish the appearance of aging face and neck skin.
(All Skin Types)
(Diane Young)
(QVC) or (www.dianeyoung.com)

8) **Firming Complex Serum**
    LeMirador

Tightens and firms the face and neck areas while reducing the appearance of fine lines and wrinkles. Helps keep skin moist and supple, improving moisture retention, elasticity and tone. Increases cell turnover, revealing a fresh new layer of smoother glowing skin.
(All Skin Types)
(LeMirador)
(QVC) or 1-800-345-1515 (www.lemiradorskincare.com)

9) **Wrinkle Firming Finish**
    Diane Young

Soften the effects of aged skin—enjoy a fresher, more toned, and younger-looking appearance with Diane Young's Wrinkle Firming Finish. The fantastic formula contains chowal mogra, a flower from India; marine botanicals like algae extract; focus serratun; bladder-wreck

extract; ascophyllium nodosum extract; amino acids lysine
and proline; and soluble collagen to hold in moisture.
(All Skin Types)
(Diane Young)
(QVC) or (www.dianeyoung.com)

10) **Awaken Younger Night Cream**
Diane Young

Good morning youth! Diane Young's Awaken Younger
Night Cream combines Chinese Botanicals with modern
technology to give your face a special treat while you sleep.
The intensive moisturizing system helps to increase the
appearance of skin firmness, plumping up lines and wrin-
kles to make them less apparent.
(All Skin Types)
(Diane Young)
(QVC) or (www.dianeyoung.com)

In order to firm the neck and décolleté areas, you will need a
skin care product made specifically for these particular areas.
The skin on the neck is thinner and will need specific skin care
products. Most women in their 30's and 40's do not treat these
areas with a moisturizer and that is a big mistake. The eye and
neck areas are the two areas that will show the signs of aging
even before the face but there is hope.

I have found products that will give you amazing results and
they are:

1) Coneflower Neckline Firmer
    Diane Young

The skin on the neck is thin, dry and has poor circulation and this condition promotes lined and sagging skin. This rich, quickly absorbed cream improves firmness, tone and texture while restoring moisture balance to the neck and décolleté areas. Within four weeks the skin's firmness will be increased by 21% and the lines and wrinkles will be decreased by 36%
(All Skin Types)
(Diane Young)
(QVC) or (www.dianeyoung.com)

2) Neck and Décolleté Cream
    Results—Joan Rivers

Sleek and Firm—Contains a powerful nutrient complex with a super-dose of exfoliating Alpha Hydroxy Acids that Cosmederm 7™ gives you. There are formulas with AHA's at levels high enough to really accomplish something, since they are buffered with COSMEDERM-7. This product firms, tones, tightens and exfoliates the neck and décolleté areas giving you a more youthful appearance.
(All Skin Types)
(Joan Rivers™)
(QVC) or (www.joanrivers.com)

3) Advanced Neck Firming Treatment
    Principal Secret

This Advanced Neck Firming Treatment with SPF 8 is a rich cream specifically formulated to combat the appear-

ance of fine lines and wrinkles that can detract from a graceful neck and smooth décolleté. Enhanced with state of the art age-defying ingredients. Matrixly and MDI complex, along with a healthy dose of anti-oxidant vitamins, hydrators and SPF 8, it helps rejuvenate and protect these delicate areas.
(All Skin Types)
(Principle Secret
c/o Guthy Renker, Dept CTJ
P.O. Box 57054 Irvine, CA 92618-7034)
(1-800-545-5595) or (www.principalsecret.com)

4)   **Neck Appeal Exfoliating**
     Diane Young

Specially designed for the delicate neck and décolleté area. Diane Young's Neck Appeal exfoliating pads contain gentle lactic acid to help smooth and soften aging skin. Use one pad every other day to help clarify skin tone, remove dead skin cells for better miniaturization and refine skin's texture by softening the appearance of lines and wrinkles. If no irritation occurs, use this product once a day.
(All Skin Types)
(Diane Young)
(QVC) or (www.dianeyoung.com)

5)   **Reverse Neck Firming Lotion Improved w/Argifirm**
     Serious Skin Care

Look your best and youngest every day with the help of Serious Skin Care's Reverse Lift Neck Firming Lotion with

improved Argifirm. This beauty treatment in a 2 oz. bottle helps hydrate, firm, tighten and streamline the appearance of sagging facial contours around the neck and jawline, leaving a visibly firmed appearance. You will love how it helps you face the world.
(All Skin Types)
(Serious Skin Care)
(Home Shopping Network)

Eye Area

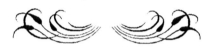

As the natural aging process progresses the eye area will thin thus causing the skin around the eye to sag. It is the loss of firmness that must be addressed in order to obtain a more youthful appearance. The delicate eye area does need special attention with products made specifically for this area. There are certain serums, gels, lotions and creams and firming products that are made especially for the skin around the eyes which is thinner and has less pores compared to the skin on the face.

The eye products I have used and recommend are:

1) **Retinol plus Vitamins—Anti-Wrinkle Firming Therapy Hydron**

Hydronamins ™ Retinol plus Vitamin C Anti-Wrinkle Firming Therapy greatly reduces the signs of aging today and slows down your skin's aging process for tomorrow. For

the first time every Hydron technology combines the proven restorative powers of Pure Retinol (Vitamin A) with the natural revitalizing capabilities of pure Vitamin C in one unique formula. It is clinically proven to reduce the appearance of lines and wrinkles while it significantly increases skin firmness and resiliency.
(All Skin Types)
(Hydron Collection)
(1-800-4HYDRON) or (www.hydron.com)

2) **Gravity Defying Eye Firming Gel**
   Sellecca Solution

This energizing eye gel leaves the delicate eye area feeling firmer and tighter. Light, oil-free formula quickly absorbs puffiness and the appearance of fine lines.
(All Skin Types)
(Sellecca Solution) (Connie Sellecca)
(www.selleccasolution.com) or (1800-866-4333)

3) **Cellular Eye Gel**
   Murad

Cooling, hydrating gel soothes, calms, firms and revitalizes the delicate eye area, reducing puffiness with aloe vera, licorice, chamomile and cucumber extracts and natural hydrating agents.
(Murad) (1-800-336-8723) or (www.murad.com)

4) **Coneflower Eyeline Firmer Treatment**
    Diane Young

    Eyeline firming complex—an eye treatment. This naturally based botanical formula helps tone, tighten, firm and instantly moisturize delicate eye area skin. Contains ingredients that will repair the eye area visibly reducing the appearance of fine lines and wrinkles.
    (All Skin Types)
    (Diane Young)
    (QVC) or (www.dianeyoung.com)

5) **Phase-Out**
    Serious Skin Care

    Phase Out is an under eye treatment from Serious Skin Care which was created with special ingredients including Vitamins C, E, K, Arnica and powerful antioxidants designed to help reduce the appearance of dark circles around the eye while evening out this sensitive area of the face.
    (All Skin Types)
    (Serious Skin Care)
    (Home Shopping Network)

6) **Reverse Lift Firming Eye Cream with**
    Argifirm
    Serious Skin Care

    Got a few sags and lines in the eye area? Help take mid-life skin back to better days—to a firmer, younger look. Reverse Lift Firming Eye Cream helps your skin look younger, thanks to our Argifirm complex, our newest in cosmetic skin care science and technology. This proprietary complex is a blend of some of the most powerful anti-aging beauty ingredients that have been shown to help firm, tighten and also help reduce the appearance of lines and wrinkles in the eye area.

(All Skin Types)

(Serious Skin Care)

(Home Shopping Network)

7) **Intensive Eye Serum—Under Eye Treatment**
    Gatineau Paris

This Kit contains 3 sets of collagen eye pads and one .51 fl. oz. of the intensive eye serum. This intensive anti-aging treatment for the eye area has a combination that helps reduce fine lines, wrinkles, puffiness and dark under eye circles. This product will give immediate results while restoring the under eye area. Results can be seen after your first application.

(All Skin Types) (Gatineau Paris) (on line)

8) **Nivea/Visage Q10 Plus Wrinkle Control**
    Eye Cream
    Nivea

This wrinkle control eye cream contains Coenzyme Q10, one of your skin's own anti-wrinkle ingredients. This eye treatment reduces the appearance of crow's feet, squint lines and wrinkles around your eyes. The ingredients in this product contain a long-term treatment.

(All Skin Types)
(Nivea) (Drug Store)

9) **Vitamin-K Dark Circle Diminished**

Vitamin K is a perfect under eye treatment. After eight weeks of daily use, you should see a dramatic difference. Use day and night. Perfect for slight discoloration.
(All Skin Types)
(Drug Store)

10) **A, C and E Eye Opener**
Kiss My Face

A botanical and vitamin enriched cream that will repair the sensitive tissues around the eye area. This product is 100% natural it contains no artificial additives.
(All Skin Types)
(Kiss My Face Corporation P.O.Box 224, Gardiner, NY 12525-0224
(www.kissmyface.com)

11) **Under Eye Renewal**
Alpha Hydrox

100% fragrance-free. Non-greasy. Advanced skin brightener evens-out dark under eye circles. Tinted-color instantly conceals dark circles. Patented TriOyygen c™ increases skin's circulation and vibrancy. Boosts production of natural collagen and new cell growth. Smoothes and protects with rich-emollients, vitamins, anti-irritants and anti-oxidants.

(All Skin Types)
(Alpha Hydrox)
(Drug Store or Neoteric Cosmetics, Inc., P.O.Box 39-S, Denver, CO 80239 or1-800-55ALPHA)
(www.alphahydrox.com)

12) **C-Circles Vanish**
Diane Young

This is a specially formulated concealer with treatment benefits. The consistency is very sheer with light diffusing properties. Contains Vitamin C, K and Licorice which will assist with the under eye skin restoration process. This product is a concealer and a treatment.
(All Skin Types)
(Diane Young)
(QVC) or (www.dianeyoung.com)

13) **A-Eye Vitamin A Eye Treatment**
A-Defiance
Serious Skin Care

Help keep your delicate eye area looking younger! Serious Skin Care brings you A-Eye (.5 oz. tube), a vitamin A cream with Retinol that helps reduce the appearance of fine lines and wrinkles around your eyes.
(Serious Skin Care)
(Home Shopping Network)

14) Glucosamine Acid-Free Skin Refining
    Eye Cream
    Serious Skin Care

This product helps to smooth fine lines and firm the delicate skin around the eye area. It contains optical diffusers
that brighten up the eye area immediately. It also helps the
eye contour look brighter, smoother and hydrated giving
you a more youthful.
(All Skin Types)
(Serious Skin Care)
(Home Shopping Network)

15) **"hope in a jar" eye and lip cream**
    Philosophy

This product promotes resilience while reducing the signs
of premature aging in the delicate eye and lip areas. This
cream contains plant extracts to help firm and protect the
skin's elastin while protecting against free radicals. Unique
blends of Vitamins C and E help to purify, moisturize, and
revitalize aged and wrinkled skin. Vitamin E helps to protect skin cells from future damage.
(All Skin Types)
(Philosophy)
(QVC) or (www.philosophy.com)

16) **Eye Complex**
    Murad

A unique, scientifically advanced eye cream that conditions
and improves the appearance of the skin around the eye

area with an exclusive lipid moisturizing formula that replenishes and improves moisture retention. Rich humectants, soothing agents and powerful, protective antioxidants combine to deliver visible results.
(Murad) mild
(1-800-336-8723) or (www.murad.com)

17) **C-No Wrinkle Eye Serum**
Serious Skin Care

This product is gentle and effective, the C-No Wrinkle Eye Serum formula is rich in Vitamin C, but also contains Vitamin K, antioxidants, progesterone and botanicals to moisturize, soothe and help reduce the appearance of fine lines, wrinkles and dark circles.
(All Skin Types)
(Serious Skin Care)
(Home Shopping Network)

18) **Performage Renewal Eye Complex**
LeMirador

A treatment for mature skin around the sensitive and delicate eye area. Contains select ingredients including Soybean Protein, Grape Seed Oil and Licorice and Mulberry Extracts to rediscover radiance and recapture smoothness. With initial use, the Performage Renewal Eye Complex will minimize the appearance of fine lines and wrinkles. Helps leave eye area seamlessly smooth and vibrant.
(All Skin Types)

(Le Mirador)

(QVC) or 1-800-345-1515 (www.lemiradorskincare.com)

19) **Critical Care Eye Cream**
Sellecca Solution

This satiny-rich eye cream provides intense hydration and soothes the fragile eye area to help reduce dark circles, puffiness and the visible signs of aging. Critical Care Eye Cream is specially formulated with a calming blend of botanicals to minimize puffiness. Leaves the eye area moisturized and looking refreshed.
(All Skin Types)
(Sellecca Solution) (Connie Sellecca)
(www.selleccasolution.com) or (1800655-4333)

20) **Nighttime Renewal for your Eyes**
Natural Advantage

This encapsulated anti-aging treatment gently delivers concentrated levels of Retinol (pure Vitamin A), Vitamins K, C, and E. and Green Tea Extract to your skin using the patented MicroRelease™ technology to help minimize the appearance of fine lines and wrinkles.
Natural Advantage)
(QVC)mild)
or (1800-276-7102) or (www.naturaladvantage.com)

21) **Miraculously Younger Eye Cream**
Diane Young

Experience the miracle of Diane Young's Dream Creams with her Miraculously Younger Eye Cream. Formulated

with multiple anti-aging technologies and botanicals, Miraculously Younger Eye Cream will help nourish and smooth the delicate skin around the eye area. Not only will it help diminish the appearance of fine lines and wrinkles, but it will also provide the skin with excellent hydration.
(All Skin Types)
(Diane Young)
(QVC) or (www.dianeyoung.com)

22) **Reclaim EyeMazing Refirming Eye Cream**
Principal Secret

You will not believe your eyes! Principal Secret Reclaim EyeMazing Eye Cream is formulated with Argireline molecular complex and other powerful ingredients to infuse the delicate skin around your eyes with long-lasting moisture. It helps fight the visible lines and wrinkles with optical diffusers for instant brightness.
(All Skin Types)
(Principle Secret
c/o Guthy Renker, Dept CTJ
P.O. Box 57054 Irvine, CA 92618-7034)
(1-800-545-5595) or (www.principalsecret.com)

23) **Glucosamine Eye Firming Gel**
Serious Skin Care

The Serious Skin Care Glucosamine Eye Firming Gel is a clear to slightly opalescent gel that visibly tightens the skin within a short time. This product is Ideal for people with

sensitive skin. The Glucosamine Eye Firming Gel is a moisturizer and eye gel firmer in one.
(All Skin Types)
(Serious Skin Care)
(Home Shopping Network)

24) **Transdermal Lipo-Peptide Complex**
Eye Patch Therapy
Spa Sciences

The first transdermal delivery system to transport a new clinically substantiated peptide complex to address the very first signs of aging on the fragile eye area. LipoPeptide Complex contains three active ingredients which restore elasticity and firmness, decrease under eye bags and discoloration, and promote lymphatic drainage to reduce puffiness. The eye area is the most mobile cutaneous surface of the body and subject to early degradation of the contours of the eyes, circulatory disorders, and product sensitivity. Test results showed that over 7-% of the panel participants with chronic under eye bags and puffiness for a period of six years or more had a highly significant decrease in the volume of their condition.
(All Skin Types)
(Spa Sciences)
(Target and Eckerd-Drug Store)(www.spasciences.com)

MASKS

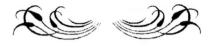

Facial masks do a variety of functions. For example, some facial masks will draw out imbedded oils, dirt and debris from the face minimizing the appearance of your pore size. Other facial masks exfoliate the skin removing the dead skin cells that have accumulated during the course of the day. Another mask will drench your skin with moisture that will hydrate your skin plumping up your fine lines and wrinkles thus lifting the area. Yet another mask will temporarily tighten your skin giving your face, neck and eye areas a lift. *Always remember that masks are temporary.*

Masks should be applied according to your skin type and the purpose of the mask. I have found masks to be beneficial for a variety of reasons.

The products which I recommend are:

1) **Triple Acting Glycolic Mask**
    Serious Skin Care

    This deep pore cleanser is used to remove oil and skin-cell debris. Helps clean pores, exfoliates surface oils while tightening the skin. This mask makes your skin feel as though it has just had a drink of hydration.
    (Serious Skin Care)
    (Home Shopping Network)

2)   **Clarifying Masque**
     Murad

Clay-based masques reduce redness, inflammation and the
severity of blemishes while healing, exfoliating, cleansing,
calming and soothing acne prone skin. Contains salicylic
acid, kaolin clay, zinc oxide, licorice, grape seed and green
tea extracts, etc. for that occasional breakout.
(Murad) (1-800-336-8723) or www.murad.com)

3)   **Results—Deep Drench Hydrating Mask**
     Joan Rivers Results

Apply once or twice a week. Deeply hydrating for thirsty
skin reducing the appearance of fine lines and wrinkles
containing a superdose of Alpha Hydroxy Acid and
Cosmederm 7™
(All Skin Types)
(Joan Rivers™)
(QVC) or (www.joanrivers.com)

4)   **Copper Collagen Infusion—**
     (Vita Peptide)
     Dr. Jeannette Graf

Give your skin the beauty treatment it deserves! Vita-
Peptide is a natural complex consisting of tiny peptide frag-
ments for effective delivery of ingredients to the skin. It
contains Artemia extract, rich in protein that works to revitalize skin. Vita-Peptide helps your skin tone, vigor, texture, and radiance. It contains copper peptides that work

with your skin's collagen to firm and plump your skin's appearance.
(All Skin Types)
(Dr. Jeannette Graf—Dermatologic Formula)
(Home Shopping Network)

5) **Honey Eye Mask**
    LeMirador

A refreshing eye mask that soothes tired eyes moisturizes, while firming and lightening the delicate skin around the eye area. It will reduce appearance of fine lines and wrinkles while moisturizing with hyaluronic acid and honey. Also contains chamomile and green tea extracts.
(All Skin Types)
(LeMirador)
(QVC) or 1-800-345-1515 (www.lemiradorskincare.com)

6) **Purifying Clay Masque**
    Murad

A refining masque with an exclusive complex that exfoliates surface skin while natural kaolin and bentonite clays gently detoxify, cleanses and absorbs impurities. Plant-derived lipids, aloe vera, allantoin and botanical extracts hydrate, soothe and renew the complexion. Contains antioxidants. Excess oil is absorbed and skin is left firmed, balanced and revitalized. Exfoliates, detoxifies and absorbs impurities while hydrating.
(Murad) (1-800-336-8723) or (www.murad.com)

7)   Silk Skin DuoMasque
     California Cosmetics

DuoMasque unites pure homeopathic remedies, natural botanicals and a multiple antioxidant defense system to help restore the supple, line free tautness of your skin. Reduces lines and wrinkles after just 3 applications. Reaches deep into our pores to pull out the impurities without stripping your skin of necessary moisture and giving you a smoother, younger looking complexion.
(California Cosmetics Corp.)
(23901 Calabasas Road, STE 2068-Calabasas, CA 91302—or (1-800-366-8243)

8)   Invisible Toning Masque
     Principal Secret

This masque should stay on for 20 minutes. If you wish, put on the masque and go shopping. After you have put it on you can not tell that you are wearing anything because it is invisible. You can even sleep in this masque for a wonderful all-night moisturizing and toning treatment. When you rinse it off, you will discover a firmer, more toned and revitalized complexion.
(All Skin Types)
(Principle Secret
c/o Guthy Renker, Dept CTJ
P.O. Box 57054 Irvine, CA 92618-7034)
(1-800-545-5595) or (www.principalsecret.com)

9) Moisture Zone Age-Controlling Hydration
    Mask
    LeMirador

    This mask deeply hydrates dry, mature skin, reducing the appearance of fine lines and wrinkles while helping to regain its youthful firmness for a smooth, soft look and feel. Use once a week for normal to dry skin, more often for very dry skin.
    (All Skin Types)
    (LeMirador)
    (QVC) or 1-800-345-1515 (www.lemiradorskincare.com)

10) Unmasked Sulfur Mask
    Serious Skin Care

    The sulfur mask contains cleansing and conditioning ingredients that help treat current skin conditions and help prevent future breakouts. The clay mask helps deep clean your pores without over drying the skin. The mask removes surface oils and the debris of dead skin cells. The active ingredient is 8% sulfur.
    (Serious Skin Care)
    (Home Shopping Network)

11) Clay Masque
    Alpha Hydrox

    This purifying clay masque (4 oz.) for normal to oily skin contains 4% Glycolic AHA with a pH 4.3 is fragrance fee containing no alcohol or oils will help with your exfoliation process while purifying your pores

(Alpha Hydrox)
(Normal to Oily Skin)
(Drug-Store)or (www.alphahydrox.com)

12) **Deep Sea: Facial Mask**
 Sumbody

Re-mineralize, revitalize and restore your glow with sea mud. High in minerals, sea mud cleanses deep from within the skin's layers and draws out impurities. This mask is a must for all types of skin. It's a deep pore cleanser, removing old oils and dirt and allowing your pores to breathe and function properly.
Sumbody is a line of skin care products that are handmade and fresh that contains all natural ingredients.
(All Skin Types)
(Sumbody) (www.sumbody.com)

13) **Chocolate Smoothie: Facial Mask**
 Sumbody

Chocolate is wonderful for softening and soothing. It's high in Linoleic Acid (the ingredient necessary for healthy, silky skin). We have added soymilk and whey to "digest" dead skin cells, colloidal oats to soothe and comfort and banana (high in Vitamin C and potassium) to moisturize. Feel the profound hydration.
Sumbody is a line of skin care products that are handmade and fresh that contains all natural ingredients.
(All Skin Types)
(Sumbody) (www.sumbody.com)

14) Blooming Masque Beauty Treatments
EcoGenics

Each EcoGenics masque will help to diminish the appearance of fine lines and wrinkles, as it helps to firm and tighten your skin giving your skin a temporary lift. The set features: (5) 0.34-oz vials, which contains extract from exotic tropical plants, as well as cucumber, chamomile, aloe and vitamins. Just pour the solution on the tablet and watch it expand with the treatment.

(All Skin Types)

(EcoGenics)(www.ecogenics.com) or (1877-372-6972)

15) Reclaim Revitalizing Youth Mask
Principal Secret

Reclaim Revitalizing Youth mask is an intense nourishment that helps to firm and clarify skin for a more luminous appearance. It is formulated with Principal Secret's breakthrough ingredient, argireline, which encourages the skin's natural renewal process while minimizing the appearance of lines and wrinkles. Use this mask twice a week after cleansing.

(All Skin Types)

(Principle Secret

c/o Guthy Renker, Dept CTJ

P.O. Box 57054 Irvine, CA 92618-7034)

(1-800-545-5595) or (www.principalsecret.com)

16) **Bee Delighted: Facial Mask**
Sumbody

What is this? More gooey fun from sumbody? This isn't just any grown up goo. It is our face reviving miracle worker (how is that for a claim?) Is your face toast? This may seem like a bread spread and tempting enough to ear, but apply our whipped honey mask to your face and feel the miracle in action. Mode with jojoba beads for a smooth, gentle exfoliation. Revitalize, repair, and restore your skin. Let go and glow! Available in raspberry, cranberry, blackberry, and apricot.
A Line of handmade, fresh and all natural ingredients.
(All Skin Types)
(Sumbody) (www.sumbody.com)

17) **It's About Time Face Mask**
Sumbody

Loaded with every natural ingredient we could find, including Vitamin C to brighten, DMAE for its time-reversing effects, and vitamins to rejuvenate and make your skin look younger, more vibrant, and incredibly youthful! One-hundred and ten percent (110%) natural ingredients bring you a face mask that is excellent for deep pore cleansing and perfect for those in need of a pore-minimizing, anti-aging, anti-oxidant miracle worker.
Sumbody is a line of skin care products that are handmade and fresh that contains all natural ingredients.
(All Skin Types)
(Sumbody) (www.sumbody.com)

18) **Fragile Eye Moisturizer**
   Hydron

   Hydron's Fragile Eye Moisturizer is formulated especially for the thin, delicate skin under and around the eye, this ultra-hydrating complex visibly smoothes eye contours, producing a 14% reduction in the appearance of fine lines and wrinkles one hour after use, and a 25% to 50% reduction after one week of daily use. Fragile Eye Moisturizer is ophthalmologist tested and approved for contact lens wearers.
   (Hydron Collection) (call 1-800-4HYDRON)
   (or www.hydron.com)

19) **Advanced Rosemary Mint Hydrating Mask**
   Principal Secret

   The Principal Secret Advanced Rosemary Mint Hydrating Mask offers the opportunity to experience the relaxation and hydration of a day spa treatment within the comfort and convenience of your home. The mask has a unique vitamin bouquet, special hydrators and exfoliators, which help provide exquisite moisture and exfoliation to your face and body in just minutes.
   (All Skin Types)
   (Principle Secret
   c/o Guthy Renker, Dept CTJ
   P.O. Box 57054 Irvine, CA 92618-7034)
   (1-800-545-5595) or (www.principalsecret.com)

20) **B-Nurture with Vitamin B Facial Mask**
Serious Skin Care

Serious Skin Care's B-Nurture is a rejuvenating facial mask that assists in removing the skin's impurities that can dull, age and contribute to a lifeless-looking complexion. Loaded with Vitamin B and naturally derived from milk, barley and honey, B-Nurture helps soften, condition and revitalize your skin.
(Serious Skin Care)
(Home Shopping Network)

21) **C-No Wrinkles Mask**
Serious Skin Care

This luxurious face conditioning mask is formulated with Vitamin C and Botanical Extracts. Use this mask to help tighten the look of your skin, minimizes your pore size, as it moisturizes and leaves your skin feeling extra soft and smooth. It also helps reduce the look of wrinkles.
(Serious Skin Care)
(Home Shopping Network)

22) **Collagen Beauty Mask**
Spa Sciences

This anti-wrinkle facial therapy product features a medical grade transdermal delivery system that transports active ingredients to the inner dermis fro improved cell respiration and turnover. The Collagen Beauty Mask is clinically proven to increase hydration while reducing sebum levels to create ideal pH levels to restore elasticity and suppleness.

Natural collagen and marine extracts provide revitalization for immediately visible results and a glowing, moiré youthful complexion. Addresses collagen depletion to prevent premature aging and wrinkling of the skin.
(Spa Sciences)
(Target and Eckerd-Drug Store)
(www.spasciences.com)

11

Procedures

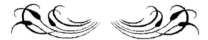

The ninth step in the restoration process is procedures. In order to accelerate the skin's renewal process, there are many procedures you can undergo at a dermatologist or cosmetic surgeon's office to enhance your appearance.

Skin renewal is the process of skin regeneration, that is, the process of taking your skin back in time as far as possible without surgery.

The type of procedure your dermatologist will recommend will be determined by the condition and coloration of your skin. If you have a few fine lines the dermatologist will most likely recommend a milder form of exfoliation while on the other hand if you have severe sun damage and deep wrinkles there will be other recommendations.

It is very important that you select the best possible doctor/surgeon for any procedure you may be contemplating. You must ask the doctor/surgeon any questions that you are anxious about. It's not surgery but most procedures today, can dramatically change your appearance. Please make sure that any doctor/surgeon you choose is board certified.

Environmental Damage

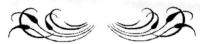

The environmental damage on the outermost layers of skin must be removed because it prevents oxygen, nutrients and moisture from reaching your healthy pink skin that is living just beneath the surface. If that isn't bad enough, those dead skin cells clinging to your top layer of skin are making your skin sag creating most of your fine lines and wrinkles and clogging your pores making them appear larger.

With all the damage being done to your skin, you will appear older if you do not start a comprehensive daily skin care routine. You can look years younger by removing layers of discolored dead skin cells just clinging to the surface of your skin.

Exfoliation

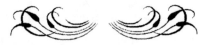

The exfoliation process is a must if you want to start taking proper care of your skin. You should exfoliate your skin in order to get the maximum benefit from any facial products you are using.

When you are in your 20's and 30's, the skin renews itself approximately once a month but when you are 40 and older, the skin's renewal process is twice as long. In other words, the dead skin cells are just clinging to your skin giving you an aged appearance. You must give nature a helping hand by exfoliating with an exfoliant as often as possible and by having some type of exfoliating procedure performed once a month.

After the age of 40, you must give nature a helping hand. That helping hand, no matter what skin type you have must be an exfoliation procedure. It does not matter which procedure you select you must select one. That procedure may be a peel, microdermabrasion, dermabrasion, laser resurfacing, ablative or nonablative, etc.

There are many exfoliation processes in which to choose. After selecting a dermatologist ask him or her to discuss all your options. Please remember research your dermatologist before making your first appointment, the responsibility of selecting a credible dermatologist is yours and yours alone.

Chemical Peels

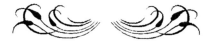

I had a few procedures which were performed by a dermatologist. Among those procedures were two chemical peels which varied in strength. Depending on the strength of the chemical peel, there may be a healing process known as down time. That down time is the time it will take for the skin to recover after the procedure. After that period of time, you will see your beautiful new skin reveal itself. That dull-looking complexion you see when you look into the mirror is years of accumulated dead skin cells and environmental damage, get rid of it.

Chemical peels use a chemical solution to remove the damaged outer layers of your skin. Chemical peels are also helpful for those individuals with facial blemishes, fine lines, wrinkles and uneven skin pigmentation and blotchiness.

Glycolic Acid Peel is an alpha hydroxy acid which will loosen dirt and debris from the pores and this peel will lighten skin discoloration and diminish fine lines and the dept of wrinkles.

Salicylic Acid Peel will help unclog follicles to help promote exfoliation. This peel will also diminish age spots.

Trichloroacitic acid (TCA) is another popular peel that is commonly used for medium depth wrinkles and uneven pig mentation.

Phenol is the strongest chemical peel and is for the most part used for deep wrinkles, skin with extreme sun damage and extreme blotchy skin tone and uneven texture. Your skin's pigmentation may be the determining factor as to whether or not this is an appropriate chemical peel for you.

All chemical peels contain some risk. Chemical peels are usually a safe procedure when performed by an experienced licensed professional.

Microdermabrasion

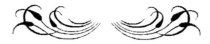

I had another procedure and that procedure was microdermabrasion. This procedure provides a deeper exfoliation than you can get from most alpha hydroxy peels. This is a noninvasive procedure also know as the "lunch time peel." Microdermabrasion is a progressive procedure using aluminum oxide crystals to remove the top layer of dead skin cells and is used to reduce fine lines, lessen the dept of your wrinkles, provide you with a more even texture and temporarily decrease the size of your pores. Microdermabrasion will remove the damaged skin and this removal will stimulate new healthy cell growth and will also stimulate collagen production.

This procedure is usually performed once every two weeks for a total of six treatments. Please also note that there is a once a month maintenance in order to maintain the turn around time you had in your 20's and 30's and that once a month removal of the surface dead skin cells will reveal a new layer of healthy skin.

If it is not cost effective for you to have this procedure once a month, then have it performed as often as possible. You need to remove all the accumulated dead skin cells from the surface of your skin that accumulate each and every minute of every day.

Laser Resurfacing

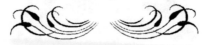

Laser resurfacing is performed by the use of a beam of laser energy that vaporizes the upper layers of damaged skin. Laser resurfacing is a carbon dioxide laser that is used to remove layers of wrinkled and/or damaged skin. The more damaged your skin, the deeper the levels of penetration, one layer at a time.

Laser resurfacing is performed if the condition of your skin needs more than a surface treatment such as a mild chemical peel or microdermabrasion. If your skin has server sun damage, deep wrinkles and sever skin discoloration this procedure will probably be recommended.

Laser resurfacing is not for everyone and that is why it is very important to seek out the best cosmetic surgeon to do this procedure. If you have brown, black or olive skin you are at risk for a pigmentation change. The surgeon will make recommendations after evaluating your skin's individual characteristics.

Do your research on any doctor that will perform any type of treatment, procedure or surgery on you. If you decide that laser resurfacing is for you, you must know the risks. Sun-damage along with the aging process does definitely contribute to the loss of resilience in your skin's tone and texture.

Fillers
(Collagen & Fat Injections)

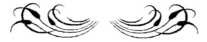

Collagen is made from cow protein and is injected into furrows and wrinkles. Collagen is usually injected between the eyebrows, the lines around the lips and the nose to mouth lines. This is a repeat procedure that will probably need to be repeated every 4 to 6 months. Allergic reactions do happen and you must be tested before having the first injection.

Fat transference is another procedure performed to plump up lines. Wrinkles and furrows. It is commonly known as a soft tissue filler. Fat is taken from your thighs, buttocks or abdomen and injected into an area that needs plumping. After a period of time, you will need more fat injected but the longevity is very lone lasting and in some cases permanent.

Botox

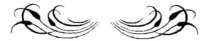

Another popular procedure is Botox injections. Botox injections will paralyze the muscle that it is injected into. Botox is a controlled toxin that is usually injected into the deep forehead lines, crows feet (lines around the eyes) and neck muscles. Botox is temporary and it usually lasts approximately 3 to 4 months before another injection is needed.

Do Your Research

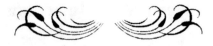

You must research any procedure you intend to have and you must also look into the background of the doctor performing the procedure. There are numerous procedures being performed and numerous persons performing those procedures do your own research, it is your face and you and you along have to live with the outcome.

There are numerous procedures being performed by dermatologists that will give you a more youthful appearance without surgery. Consult with a dermatologist, he or she will guide you in the right direction. Ultimately, the decision is yours.

If you do not want to have cosmetic surgery you can select from the numerous procedures being performed today, the choice is your. My choice, at least for now, is to grow older gracefully. In the future, I may change my outlook on this particular aspect of my life or I may stand firm, the choice is mine.

When selecting a dermatologist, make sure that he or she has performed a particular procedure repeatedly. Select a doctor who will take the time to listen to your concerns and answer your questions and make sure that he or she thoroughly explains the procedure. Check his or her credentials, ask questions. Ask if the doctor is continuing his or her medical education to keep up with all the new techniques and procedures within his or her field of expertise. Ask your dermatologist for before and after photos. It is your responsibility to do the research. Ask for references, ask all the questions you are anxious about and read all the material you can on any procedure you may be interested in undergoing. The individual you select to perform any type of procedure will not mind answering any and all the questions you have. A satisfied patient is a walking-talking advertisement.

Do not get the phone book out and pick one, ask friends and family members and your family physician for recommendations.

Whatever you decide to do in order to make you feel better about yourself, just do it. Some people care about their appearance while others do not. This is your decision! It is up to you.

Approximately three-quarters of the women today would rather use creams as opposed to cosmetic surgery and those creams are out there and the cost of the creams, serums, vitamins, etc. do not have to be out-of-reach for the average working-class woman. Knowing your skin type and your skin's needs will help you select the best skin care products for you.

If you decide that surgery is what you want, you will still need creams, lotions, gels, vitamins, etc. to keep your skin in the best possible condition. Your skin should be kept in exceptional condition in order to achieve a more youthful and healthy appearance. A surgeon can lift your skin but what condition will your skin be in, that choice is up to you.

If you elect to have any type of cosmetic surgery, below I have listed a few that may interest you and they are:

Forehead lift/browlift—Is a process where the top third of your face is lifted.

Upper and/or lower eyelid surgery/eyelid tuck—A process where your eye area is lifted.

Traditional Facelift—Your entire face, from your forehead to your chin is lifted.

Mid-facelift—A process where your cheek area is lifted.

Neck lift or liposuction—A process where your neck will be liposuctioned, incisions are made and the skin is lifted giving your neck area a softer and smoother appearance.

Dermaplaning—Dermaplaning is a procedure not a surgery.

Dermaplaning

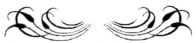

Dermaplaning is a procedure that has been performed in Japan for years. It is a simple procedure that must always be performed by a doctor.

The qualified doctor will take a surgical scalpel and scrape off layers of skin. Dermaplaning will exfoliate the skin if you have problems with uneven skin tone and texture, superficial line or superficial wrinkles. With this resurfacing technique there are no chemicals used and each session is approximately 20 minutes. It is advised that the treatment be performed once a month for three consecutive months. Dermaplaning does provide a new non-invasive option for those looking for a fresh new look.

With any surgery or procedure, please know that there are risks and you must be an informed consumer. Learn all you can about the procedure and the person performing the procedure.

We have so many choices that your choices are almost endless. Whether you decide to have a procedure or surgery the research is up to you. Do not rely completely on any one person. Ask your family physician, go to the library and go on-line, the knowledge you have is through research.

If you would like to find a qualified dermatologist you should call the American Society for Dermatology (ASDS) at 1-800-441-2737 during weekday or visit the web site at www.asds-net.org. If you have decided on cosmetic surgery, you should call the American Society of Plastic Surgeon at 1-888-475-2784 during the weekday or visit the Web site at www.plasticsurgery.org.

You must do the research. When you are looking for a house, what do the experts say "location, location, location." When looking for a dermatologist or cosmetic and/or plastic surgeon, what do the experts say "research, research, and more research." That research is ultimately up to you and no one else.

12

Spa Treatment

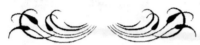

Take time out from your busy schedule and go to a spa. A trip to a day spa is well worth your time. There are so many types of facials to choose from and the benefits are immediate, and extremely beneficial. When you can walk out of a spa relaxed and with a healthy glow, it is well worth your time and money.

Of course, if you wish, you may steam clean your face with a steam machine or if you wish, you can fill your sink with very hot water and after placing a towel over your hair and another towel over your head and the sink, thus preventing the steam from escaping, you can now relax for approximately three to five minutes while the steam opens your pores.

After you have opened your pores with steam, washed your face with an exfoliating product by hand or by machine, make sure that every part of your face and neck (front and back) have been exfoliated, close your pores with cool water or a cool mist.

There is a facial steamer on the market today that not only uses hot steam to open your pores but it also has a second function that emits a cool mist to close your pores.

If you give yourself a facial at home the process should take no longer than fifteen to twenty minutes and that fifteen to twenty minutes you have taken to steam clean, exfoliate and moisturize you face is time well spent and a bonus, you will be more relaxed. After the steam facial, you are ready to put your skin care products on from the thinnest to the thickest.

Essential Oils

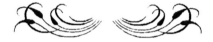

There are different essential oils that you can put into your facial steam machine or your sink to enhance your facial.

As always, with any new skin care product, such as essential oils, consult with a skin care specialist. Some essential oils cannot be used when you are pregnant or if you have a skin condition or breathing condition.

All essential oils must be tested on an inconspicuous area of the skin and most essential oils must be diluted with carrier oils. To know the proper amount to use, please always ask a specialist. Most essential oils cannot be placed directly onto the skin; they must be combined with other oils such as carrier oils. Some essentials oils can burn the skin. Some of the essential oils used in skin care are mentioned below.

Experiment with caution and do your homework before applying any new products on your skin.

Oily/Acne prone Skin

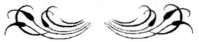

Chamomile—calming, balancing
Tea Tree—antibacterial, antiseptic
Rose—refines pores
Lavender—soothing, calming
Lemongrass—calming, balancing
Rosemary—purifying, clarifying

Dry Skin/Mature

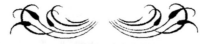

Bergamot—soothing, calming
Lavender—soothing, calming
Patchouli—grounding, clarifying
Rosemary—purifying, clarifying
Geranium—balancing, regenerative
Fennel—tonic, balancing
Peppermint—calming, balancing.

Combination/Normal Skin

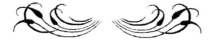

Geranium—balancing, regenerative
Bergamot—soothing, calming
Lavender—soothing, calming
Almond—protects and nourishes, "carrier oil"
Apricot—revitalize dry skin carrier oil
Rosemary—purifying, clarifying

Never use essential oils full strength on your skin always use a filler oil to mix with your essential oils.

When purchasing essential oils, ask the company representative which filler oils would be best for your type skin and be sure to tell them what you intend to do with the oils so that they can guide you in the right direction.

There are so many essential oils in which to choose from just remember to do your research and test any new product on an inconspicuous area near your ear or on your jaw line.

Please remember when you are steaming your face with an essential oil that you will also be breathing in that oil, so take every precaution and ask your physician if the oil you have selected can be inhaled. The oil that you have selected may be something that you should not be breathing in so be careful, do your research.

After your day spa or your at home spa experience you will look and feel more relaxed and refreshed and yes, the best part, what a glow.

If you have the time or even if you don't, find the time to go to the day spa and indulge yourself, you deserve it, we all do.

Think of a facial as a thorough spring cleaning. That thorough cleaning will include a surface cleaning, as well as a deep pore cleaning, a mild exfoliation, toning and moisturizing.

There are many types of facials and just to mention as few:

Acne Facial
Anti-Aging Facial
European Seaweed Facial
Natural Facial
Rosacea Treatment Facial
Vitamin Facial
AHA treatment Facial
Aromatherapy Facial
Hydrating Facial
Oxygen Therapy Facial
Steaming Facial

There are numerous facials to choose from and most spas have their own names for them. Some names are very exotic and some names are straight to the point.

Upon making an appointment with your favorite day spa, ask for a one-on-one consultation with a spa consultant or professional facialist.

During the consultation, the skin care professional should analyze you skin and inform you as to which facial would be most beneficial. The spa consultant should examine your skin under a magnifying glass and you should also be asked about your life style such as your exposure to the elements and your dietary habits. From this meeting, the consultant will be able to guide you in the right direction regarding which facial or facials are best for your particular needs.

A good basic facial would be to have your face thoroughly steamed which would free your skin of all dirt, pollution and debris and in doing so, your pores will appear smaller. After the cleaning, you should have an exfoliating process and before leaving the comfort of the spa, ask for a hydrating moisturizer and that in my estimation, is a perfect facial. Are you ready? If you are, it is time for you to find the perfect day spa for your very own customized facial.

A spa facial will cost approximately $50 to $175 per visit depending on what type of facial you choose. Just pick up the telephone and call a spa near you and ask what type of services they provide and the cost for each type of facial. More often then not, they will be happy to send you information regarding their services and prices.

If you decide to go to the spa just to have a good thorough cleaning the relaxation will do wonders for you mentally as well as physically. You will not only look healthier and more youthful but you will be more relaxed. We deserve to pamper ourselves and whether that pampering is at home or at the spa, you deserve to be pampered and so do I.

Humidifiers/Moisture

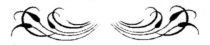

In the winter months, your home and office are usually air tight and with the artificial heat surrounding you, your skin will need extra moisture. You should be getting moisture from your diet and your skin care products as well as your daily intake of water but do not forget that putting moisture into the air is also important.

Go to your local beauty supply store, department store or drug store and purchase a humidifier. If you do not want the maintenance of a humidifier, place containers of water throughout your house and if they are pretty containers no one will know that they are filled with water. If you do this small step your skin will be more hydrated thus giving your skin a more youthful look. Just remember to change the water and clean the containers often.

13

Homemade Skin Care Recipes

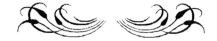

The tenth and last step in the restoration process is to use products and/or ingredients that you may already have in your own home. From my home to your home and yes, I have tried them all and have found them to be effective.

Please always remember if you have delicate or sensitive skin, test an area behind the ear or near your jaw bone to see if you are allergic to any new product whether the product is nature or not you may have an allergic reaction. Always take preventive measures when testing any new ingredient.

I have provided you with a list of my favorites:

Oily Skin

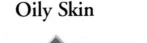

Oily skin is caused by over-active glands. You can reduce the production of oil by exfoliating and steaming your face.

Some of the many homemade facial treatments are:

Sugar Cleanser (exfoliating)—After taking off your makeup and cleansing your skin, take a small amount of sugar, yes ordinary table sugar. Add a small amount of water to make a paste like consistency. Rub the mixture on the face, eye and neck areas. This process will help to loosen the dead skin cells on the outer layer of skin so that the dead skin cells come off easier. When using any abrasive be gentle around the eye area. Rinse with warm water then splash on cool water. Moisturize with your favorite moisturizer.
Ingredients: sugar.

Baking Soda Cleanser and/or Mask (exfoliating)—Combine baking soda and water together and cleanse your skin. After cleansing combine the baking soda and water making a paste. Apply the mixture to your face and neck areas as a mask for 10 minutes to exfoliate. Remove with warm water, splash with cool water. Moisturize as usual. Polishes the skin giving you a healthy glow.
Ingredients: Baking Soda.

Salt or Sugar Cleanser and Olive Oil Mask (exfoliating)—Place a tablespoon of salt or sugar in the palm of your hand then mix in some olive oil (cosmetic olive oil), just enough to make a paste. Rub the mixture into your face, neck and décolleté areas. Make sure that you rub this mixture in an upward circular motion for approximately 1 minute. Let the mixture sit on those areas for approximately 30 minutes. Rub in again then rinse with warm water and splash with cool water. Moisturize as usual. Ingredients: Salt, Sugar & Olive Oil.

Almond Meal Cleanser (exfoliating)—Combine 4 tablespoons or almond meal, 2 tablespoons or Jojoba oil, 3 tablespoons of honey 4 drops of Peppermint oil and 1 drop of lemon oil in a glass bowl. Combine and mix the ingredients thoroughly. After you have washed your face with warm water scrub your face with this exfoliating scrub. Rinse with cool water. Moisturize as usual. Note: This scrub is not for sensitive or dry skin. Ingredients: Almond Meal, jojoba oil, honey, peppermint oil & lemon oil.

Fruit Toner (skin brightener)—Squeeze 1 whole lemon or 1 whole lime or you may use both. Add the juice to 1 cup of water then put the mixture into a spray bottle and use as a daily toner, do not wash off. Discard after 2 weeks. Moisturize as usual. Ingredients: Fresh lemon & lime.

Tea Toner (lackluster skin)—Combine 1 decaffeinated organic green tea bag and 1 decaffeinated chamomile tea bag into a cup of boiling water. After 10 minutes remove the tea bags. Put the

mixture into a spray bottle, add one cup of cool water and place the mixture into the refrigerator. Use daily as a toner. Do not wash off. Discard after 2 weeks. Moisturize as usual.
Note: Contains powerful antioxidants to repair environmentally damaged skin.
Ingredients: Decaffeinated organic green tea, decaffeinated chamomile tea.

Vinegar Toner (restores the pH balance)—Combine 1/4 cup of apple cider vinegar and 3 cups of water. Put the mixture into a spray bottle. Keep in refrigerator. Use daily as a toner. Do not wash off. Discard after two weeks. Moisturize as usual.
Ingredients: Apple cider vinegar.

Pineapple Mask (exfoliating)—Place a fresh pineapple into a juicer then put the juice on your face, neck and eye areas for 30 minutes or longer. A good exfoliant. Remove with warm water, splash with cool water. Moisturize as usual.
Ingredients: Fresh pineapple.

Almond Meal Mask (exfoliating)—Mix almond meal with enough water for a paste like consistency. Put the almond meal on your pores for 10 to 30 minutes as a mask. After removing the mask with tepid water, mix a small amount of almond meal and water and wash you face, neck and eye areas in a circular and upward direction to remove any dead skin cells. When using an abrasive around the eye area, continue with caution. Rinse with warm water, splash with cool water. Moisturize as usual.
Ingredients: Almond meal.

Tomato, Avocado & Fruit Mask (brightens the complexion)— Use ½ of a tomato, 1 avocado, ½ lemon and ½ lime. After removing the pit from the avocado place the tomato and avocado in a juicer or blender until mixture is a smooth consistency. Empty the finished product into a bowl and add the juice of the lemon and lime until blended. Place the mask on your face and neck areas for approximately 10 to 30 minutes. This mask will brighten you complexion. Moisturize as usual.
Ingredients: Fresh tomato, avocado, lemon, lime.

Sea Salt and Buttermilk Mask (exfoliates & introduces extra calcium & protein to the skin's cells)—Add sea salt to buttermilk (paste like consistency) then put the mixture on the areas of your face that contain enlarged pores and massage for approximately 2 minutes. After cleansing with this combination use the remaining mixture as a mask and leave on for 10 minutes or longer. Then wash with warm water, splash with cool water. Moisturize as usual.
Ingredients: Sea salt & buttermilk.

Avocado Mask (hydrating)—Combine the juice of 1 ripe avocado, 1 tablespoon of plain yogurt, 1 tablespoon of olive oil (cosmetic olive oil) or almond oil and 1 tablespoon of lemon or lime juice. Put the mixture on your face, neck and eye areas for 30 minutes. Remove with warm water, splash with cool water. Moisturize as usual.
Ingredients: Fresh avocado, plain yogurt, olive oil, almond oil, lemon & lime.

Strawberry Mask (exfoliates & refreshes the skin while reducing redness)—Cut a strawberry in half. Rub the juice onto the face and neck areas. Leave on the juice for 30 minutes re-applying every 10 minutes. Remove with warm water, splash with cool water. Moisturize as usual.
Ingredients: Fresh strawberries.

Strawberry & Honey Mask (exfoliates & refreshes the skin while reducing redness/hydrates)—Mash 10 strawberries and fold in 3 tablespoons of honey. Apply the mixture to your face and neck areas, let the mixture stay on those area for 20 minutes. Remove with warm water, splash with cool water. Moisturize as usual.
Ingredients: Fresh strawberries & Honey.

Lemon/Lime & Egg Mask (firm & tighten)—Combine 1/4 cup of lemon or lime juice and 1 egg white slightly beaten. Put the mixture on your face and neck areas for 30 minutes. Your skin will be firmer. Remove with warm water, splash with cool water. Moisturize as usual.
Ingredients: Fresh lemon, lime & egg.

Honey, Almond Oil & Egg Mask (hydrating)—Combine 2 tablespoons of honey, 3 drops of almond oil and 1 egg yolk. Put the mixture on your face and neck areas for 30 minutes. This is a great hydrator Remove with warm water, splash with cool water. Moisturize as usual.
Ingredients: Honey, almond oil & egg.

Cucumber & Lemon/Lime Mask (more even skin tone)—Mix 1 teaspoon of lime or lemon juice with 1 teaspoon of cucumber juice and a few drops of rose water. Put the mixture on the face and neck areas. Leave on for 30 minutes. More even skin tone. Remover with warm water, splash with cool water. Moisturize as usual.
Ingredients: Fresh cucumber, lime, lemon cucumber & rose water.

Tomato Mask (lightens skin & fades spots)—Slice a tomato, spread the slice of tomato onto your face every 15 minutes for 30 minutes then remove with water, splash with cool water. Moisturize as usual.
Ingredients: Fresh tomato.

Tomato Juice Mask (lightens skin & fades spots)—Combine 1 tablespoon of tomato juice and 1/2 teaspoon of lime or lemon juice. Put the mixture on your face and neck areas for 30 minutes. Remove with warm water, splash with cool water. Moisturize as usual.
Ingredients: Tomato juice, fresh lime or lemon.

Yogurt & Fruit Mask (smooth out wrinkles & fades age spots)—Combine 2 tablespoons of brewer's yeast, 1/2 teaspoon of fresh lemon juice or lime juice and enough yogurt to make a loose paste. Put on face and neck, where oily, for 30 minutes. Remove with warm water, splash with cool water. Moisturize as usual.
Ingredients: Brewer's yeast, lemon, lime & yogurt.

Avocado Mask (boost your skin's collagen & fades imperfections)—Combine 1 avocado, 1 cooked carrot into a bowl whip into a smooth consistency then add 3 tablespoons of honey ½ cup of heavy cream and 1 beaten egg then blend all ingredients until smooth. Gently fold 1 drop of lemon oil and 1 drop of orange oil into the mixture. Place ½ of the ingredients onto the face and neck areas leave mask on for approximately 20 to 30 minutes, rinse with cool water. Place the remaining portion into refrigerator in an air tight container and use the remainder portion the next day but keep this mask no longer then 1 day in your refrigerator. This mask will boost your skin's collagen and will help fade imperfections. This combination should make two masks. You should always blend oils such as orange or lemon before using in any configuration. Never use nature oils directly onto the eye, face or neck areas.

Ingredients: Fresh avocado, carrot, honey, heavy cream, egg, orange oil & lemon oil.

Dry Skin

Dry skin is usually caused when the skin does not produce enough sebum in order to maintain an oily surface.

Some of the many homemade facial remedies are:

Oatmeal Cleanser (hydrates & softens) place old fashion Oatmeal into the foot portion of an old nylon stocking then

place the nylon under hot running water until oats are soft. Then rub the oats still in the nylon onto the face and neck areas for 1 to 3 minutes then discard.
Ingredients: Oatmeal.

Tea Toner (lackluster skin)—Combine 1 decaffeinated organic green tea bag and 1 decaffeinated chamomile tea bag into one cup of boiling water. After 10 minutes remove the tea bags. Put the mixture into a spray bottle. Add 1 cup of cool water into the mixture and refrigerate. Use daily as a toner. Discard after 2 weeks.
Note: Contains powerful antioxidants to repair environmentally damaged skin.
Ingredients: Decaffeinated organic green tea & decaffeinated chamomile tea.

Cucumber, Honey & Fruit Toner (complexion brightener)—Place 1 medium cucumber into a juicer then take that juice and place it into a glass container add 2 teaspoons of honey and the juice of ¼ lemon into the same container then shake ingredients until blended. Put the mixture onto a cotton ball then put the mixture onto your face and neck area. Leave mixture on the face as your daily toner, then moisturize. You can leave this mixture in the refrigerator for approximately seven days.
Ingredients: Fresh cucumber, honey & lemon.

Cucumber Toner (soothes and calms skin)—Put a cucumber into a juicer. Put the juice in the refrigerator over night. Add 1 cup of cool water. Spray onto face every day for a nourishing

toner. Do not wash off, this is your daily toner. Discard after two weeks. Moisturize as usual.
Ingredients: Fresh cucumber.

Honey and Almond Oil Mask (hydrating)—Combine 2 tablespoons of honey and 2 tablespoons of almond oil. Put the mixture onto the face and neck areas for 15 to 20 minutes or longer if you wish. Remove with warm water, splash with cool water. What a glow. Moisturize as usual.
Ingredients: Honey & almond oil.

Honey, Almond Oil & Oil of Rose Mask (hydrating)—Combine 4 tablespoons of honey, 4 tablespoons of sweet almond oil and 8 drops of essential oil of rose. Put on face and neck areas for 30 minutes. Remove with warm water, splash with cool water. Moisturize as usual.
Ingredients: Honey, sweet almond oil & essential oil of rose.

Avocado, Egg, Yogurt and Olive Oil Mask (hydrating)—Combine the juice from 1 ripe avocado, 1 egg yolk, 1 tablespoon of plain yogurt and 1 tablespoon of olive oil (cosmetic olive oil). Put on face, neck and eye areas for 30 minutes to one hour. Remove with warm water, splash with cool water. Moisturize as usual.
Ingredients: Fresh avocado, egg, yogurt & olive oil.

Olive Oil Mask (hydrating)—Put olive oil (cosmetic olive oil) on your face and neck areas overnight at least twice a week. This

will moisturize and nourish the skin. Wash off in the morning. Moisturize as usual.
Ingredients: Olive oil.

Olive Oil & Lemon/Lime Mask (hydrating)—Combine 1 tablespoon of lemon juice and/or lime juice and 1 tablespoon of olive oil (cosmetic olive oil). Put the mixture on face and neck areas for 30 minutes. Remove with warm water, splash with cool water. Moisturize as usual.
Ingredients: Fresh lemon, lime & olive oil.

Honey, Olive Oil, Egg and Vitamin E Mask (hydrating)— Combine 1 teaspoon honey, 1 teaspoon olive oil (cosmetic olive oil) 1 egg yolk and 1/4 teaspoon of Vitamin E oil or use the liquor from 3 Vitamin E capsules. Put the mixture onto face and neck areas. Leave on face and neck areas for 30 minutes. Remove with warm water, splash with cool water. Moisturize as usual.
Ingredients: Honey, olive oil, egg & vitamin E.

Honey, Olive Oil & Egg Mask (hydrating)—Combine 1 teaspoon of honey, 1 teaspoon of olive oil (cosmetic olive oil) and 1 egg yolk. After you have combined the above ingredients add enough oatmeal to make a paste. Leave the mixture on face and neck areas for 30 minutes. Remove with warm water, splash with cool water. Moisturize as usual.
Ingredients: Honey, olive oil & egg.

Egg, Lime & Olive Oil Mask (hydrating)—Mix 1 egg yolk, 1 tablespoon of fresh lime juice and 1 tablespoon of olive oil

(cosmetic olive oil). Put the mixture on the face and neck areas for 30 minutes. Remove with warm water, splash with cool water. Moisturize as usual.
Ingredients: Egg, fresh lime & olive oil.

Banana Mask (softens and moisturizes)—Mash a banana then apply to face, neck and eye areas for 30 minutes. Remove with warm water, splash with cool water. Moisturize as usual.
Ingredients: Fresh banana.

Banana & Honey Mask (softens and moisturizes)—Mash a banana and add 2 tablespoons of honey. Mix to a smooth but not runny consistency then apply to your face, neck and eye areas for 30 minutes. Remove with warm water, splash with cool water. Moisturize as usual.
Ingredients: Fresh banana & honey.

Peach & Honey Mask (exfoliates and increases the rate of new cell growth)—Combine the juice of 1 peach and 1 tablespoon of honey. Put mixture onto the face and neck areas for 30 minutes. Remove with warm water, splash with cool water. Moisturize as usual.
Ingredients: Fresh peach & honey.

Honey, Almond Oil & Egg Mask (hydrating)—Combine 2 tablespoons of honey, 3 drops of almond oil and two egg yolks. Put the mixture on the face and neck areas for 30 minutes.

Remove with warm water, splash with cool water. Moisturize as usual.

Ingredients: Honey, almond oil & egg.

Avocado and More Mask (boosts collagen production and fades age spots)—Combine 1 avocado, 1 cooked carrot into a bowl whip into a smooth consistency then add 3 tablespoons of honey ½ cup of heavy cream and 1 beaten egg then blend all ingredients until smooth. Gently fold 1 drop of lemon oil and 1 drop of orange oil into the mixture. Place ½ of the ingredients onto the face and neck areas leave mask on for approximately 20 to 30 minutes, rinse with cool water. Place the remaining portion into refrigerator in an air tight container and use the remainder portion the next day but keep this mask no longer then 1 day in your refrigerator. This mask will boost your skin's collagen and will help fade imperfections. This combination should make two masks. You should always blend oils such as orange or lemon before using in any configuration. Never use nature oils directly onto the eye, face or neck areas.

Ingredients: Fresh avocado & carrot, honey, heavy cream, egg, lemon oil, & orange oil.

Peaches and Cream Nighttime Mask (exfoliates & increases the rate of new cell growth)—Combine the juice of 1 peach, place the peach in a juicer then add 4 tablespoons of heavy cream. Put the combined mixture on face, neck and eye areas over night. Wash off in the morning, Moisturize as usual. Do this three time a week. For a peaches and cream complexion.

Ingredients: Fresh peach & heavy cream.

Rosewater & Jojoba Oil Nighttime Moisturizer (hydrating)—Combine 2 tablespoons of Rosewater and 2 tablespoons of Jojoba oil. Put the mixture on your face and neck areas over night at least twice a week. Moisturize as usual.
Ingredients: Rosewater & jojoba oil.

Normal/Combination Skin

Normal skin produces an average amount of sebum and is neither oily nor dry.

Some of the many homemade facial remedies are:

Sugar Cleanser (exfoliating)—After taking off your makeup and cleansing your skin, take a small amount of sugar, yes ordinary table sugar. Add a small amount of water. Rub the mixture on the face, eye and neck areas. This process will help to loosen the dead skin cells on the very top layer of skin so that they come off easier. Rinse with warm water then splash on cool water, moisturize with your favorite moisturizer.
Ingredients: Sugar.

Baking Soda Cleanser and/or Mask (exfoliating)—Combine baking soda and water to cleanse your skin. After cleansing combine the baking soda and water making a paste like consistency. Apply the mixture to your face and neck areas as a mask

for 10 minutes to polish the skin. Remove with warm water, splash with cool water. Moisturize as usual.
Ingredients: Baking soda.

Almond Meal Cleanser and Mask (exfoliating)—Put almond meal with enough water for a paste like consistency. Put the almond meal on your pores for 10 minutes. Combine a small amount of almond meal and mix with water. Wash you face, neck and eye area in a circular upward motion. Use a gentle touch around the eye area. This technique will rid you skin of dead skin cells. Rinse with warm water, splash with cool water. Moisturize as usual.
Ingredients: Almond meal

Salt and Olive Oil Cleanser and/or Mask (exfoliating)—Place a tablespoon of salt or sugar in the palm of your hand then blend in some olive oil (cosmetic olive oil), just enough to make a paste. Rub the mixture into your face, neck and décolleté areas. Make sure that you rub this mixture in an upward circular motion. After approximately one-minute, let the mixture sit on those areas for approximately 10 to 30 minutes. Rub in once again then rinse off with warm water, splash with cool water. Makes a great Exfoliant. Moisturize as usual.
Ingredients: Salt, sugar & olive oil.

Almond meal, Jojoba Oil and Honey Cleanser (exfoliating)—Combine 4 tablespoons or almond meal, 2 tablespoons or Jojoba oil, 3 tablespoons of honey, 4 drops of Peppermint oil and 1 drop of lemon oil in a glass bowl. Combine and mix the ingredients thoroughly. After you have washed your face with warm water scrub your face with this exfoliating scrub. Rinse with cool water. Moisturize as usual. Note: This scrub is not for sensitive or dry skin.

Ingredients: Almond meal, jojoba oil, honey, peppermint oil & lemon oil.

Tea Toner (lackluster skin)—Combine 1 decaffeinated organic green tea bag and 1 decaffeinated chamomile tea bag into one cup of boiling water. After 10 minutes remove the tea bags. Put the mixture into a spray bottle. Add 1 cup of cool water into the mixture and refrigerate. Use daily as a toner. Do not wash off. Contains powerful antioxidants to repair environmentally damaged skin.

Ingredients: Decaffeinated organic green tea & decaffeinated chamomile tea.

Ingredients: Green tea & chamomile tea.

Cucumber, Honey & Lemon Toner (complexion brightener)—Place 1 medium cucumber into a juicer then take that juice and place it into a glass container add 2 teaspoons of honey and the juice of ¼ lemon into the same container then shake ingredients until blended. Put the mixture onto a cotton ball then put the mixture onto your face and neck area. Leave mixture on the face as your daily toner, then moisturize. You can leave this mixture in the refrigerator for approximately seven days.

Ingredients: Fresh cucumber & lemon & honey.

Pineapple Mask (exfoliating)—Put a fresh pineapple into a juicer. Use the juice from the pineapple on your face, neck and eye areas for 30 minutes or longer. Remove with warm water, splash with cool water. Moisturize as usual.
Ingredients: Fresh pineapple.

Honey & Sweet Almond Oil Mask (hydrating)—Combine 4 tablespoons of honey, 4 tablespoons of sweet almond oil and 8 drops of essential oil of rose. Put the mixture on face and neck areas for 30 minutes. Remove with warm water, splash with cool water. Moisturize as usual.
Ingredients: Honey, sweet almond oil & essential oil of rose.

Tomato, Avocado & Lemon/Lime Mask (brightens the complexion)—Combine ½ of a tomato, 1 avocado, ½ lemon and ½ lime then after removing the pit from the avocado, place the tomato and avocado in a juicer or blender until mixture is a smooth consistency. Empty the finished product into a bowl and add the juice of the lemon and lime until blended. Place the mask on your face and neck areas for approximately 10 to 30 minutes. This mask will brighten you complexion. Moisturize as usual.
Ingredients: Fresh avocado, tomato, lemon & lime.

Banana & Honey Mask (softens & moisturizes)—Mash a banana and add 2 tablespoons of honey. Mix to a smooth but not runny consistency, and then apply to face, neck and eye areas for 30 minutes. Remove with warm water, splash with cool water. Moisturize as usual.
Ingredients: Fresh banana & honey.

Sea Salt & Buttermilk Mask (exfoliates & introduces extra calcium & protein to the skin's cells)—Add sea salt to buttermilk (paste like consistency) then put the mixture on the areas of your face that contain enlarged pores and massage for approximately 2 minutes. After cleansing with this combination use the remaining mixture as a mask and leave on for 10 minutes or longer. Then wash with warm water, splash with cool water. Moisturize as usual.
Ingredients: Sea sale & buttermilk.

Honey & Almond Oil Mask (hydrating)—Combine 2 tablespoons of honey and 2 tablespoons of almond oil to face and neck areas for 30 minutes to 1 hour. Remove with warm water, splash with cool water. What a glow. Moisturize as usual.
Ingredients: Honey & almond oil.

Milk, Honey and Lemon/Lime Mask (exfoliating)—Combine 1 tablespoon of milk, 1 tablespoon of honey and 3 drops of lemon juice or lime juice. Put the mixture on face, neck and eye areas for 30 minutes. A perfect exfoliant. Remove with warm water, splash with cool water. Moisturize as usual.
Ingredients: Milk, honey & fresh lemon & lime.

Avocado & More Mask (boosts your skin's collagen production)—Combine 1 avocado, 1 cooked carrot into a bowl whip into a smooth consistency then add 3 tablespoons of honey ½ cup of heavy cream and 1 beaten egg then blend all ingredients until smooth. Gently fold 1 drop of lemon oil and 1 drop of orange oil into the mixture. Place ½ of the ingredients onto the face and neck areas leave mask on for approximately 20 to 30 minutes, rinse with cool water. Place the remaining portion into refrigerator in an air tight container and use the remainder portion the next day but keep this mask no longer then 1 day in your refrigerator. This mask will boost your skin's collagen and will help fade imperfections. This combination should make two masks. You should always blend oils such as orange or lemon before using in any configuration. Never use nature oils directly onto the eye, face or neck areas.

Ingredients: Fresh avocado & carrot, honey, heavy cream, egg, lemon oil & orange oil.

Strawberry & Honey Mask (exfoliates & refreshes the skin while reducing redness/hydrates)—Mash 10 strawberries and fold in 3 tablespoons of honey. Apply the mixture to your face and neck areas, let the mixture stay on those area for 20 minutes. Remove with warm water, splash with cool water. Moisturize as usual.

Ingredients: Fresh strawberries & honey.

Papaya Mask (exfoliating)—Put a pitted and peeled papaya in a juicer. Put the juice on your eye, face and neck areas for 30 minutes. Remove with warm water, splash with cool water. This papaya make will slough off dead skin cells. Moisturize as usual.

Ingredients: Fresh papaya.

Apricot Mask (restores the skin's elasticity)—Put a pitted and peeled apricot in a juicer. Put the juice of your eye, neck and face areas for 30 minutes. Remove with warm water, splash with

cool water. This mask will held restore the skin's elasticity. Moisturize as usual.
Ingredients: Fresh apricot.

Bael Fruit Extract & Honey Mask (improves skin's elasticity)—Combine 2 tablespoons of Bael fruit extract and 1 tablespoon of honey to your face, neck and eye areas for 30 minutes. Remove with warm water, splash with cool water. This mask will held improves the skin's elasticity. Moisturize as usual.
Ingredients: Bael fruit extract & honey.

Milk Mask (exfoliating)—Put whole milk on your face, neck and eye areas for 20 to 30 minutes. Rinse warm water, splash with cool water. This mask is a great exfoliant. Moisturize as usual.
Ingredients: Milk.

Egg Mask (tightens the skin)—Use 1 egg white—slightly beaten, put on face, neck and eye areas. Leave on for 15 to 20 minutes. Tightens the skin. Wash off with warm water then splash with cool water before moisturizing.
Ingredients: Egg.

Pineapple, Papaya & Honey Mask (exfoliating and hydrating)—Combine 1 cup of fresh pineapple, 1/2 cup of fresh papaya, 2 tbs. of honey—puree papaya and pineapple then add honey. Mix ingredients together. Depending on your skin type, put on face and neck areas 5 minutes (oily skin) to 15 to 30

minutes (dry or mature skin). Rinse with warm water, splash on cool water then moisturize.
Ingredients: Honey & fresh pineapple & papaya.

Olive Oil & Lemon/Lime Mask (hydrating)—Combine 1 tablespoon of lime juice, 1 tablespoon of lemon juice and 1 tablespoon of olive oil (cosmetic olive oil). Put on face and neck areas for 30 minutes. Remove with warn water, splash with cool water. Moisturize as usual.
Ingredients: Olive oil, fresh lime & lemon.

Oatmeal, Olive Oil and Egg Mask (hydrating)—Combine 1/2 cup of uncooked instant oatmeal, 1 teaspoon of olive oil (cosmetic olive oil) and 1 egg yolk. Leave on face, neck and eye areas for 30 minutes. Hydrates the skin. Remove with warm water, splash with cool water.
Ingredients: Oatmeal, olive oil & egg.

Strawberry, Papaya, Peach & Honey Mask (exfoliates & refreshes the skin while reducing redness/hydrates)—Combine 3 strawberries, 1/4 cup of mashed papaya, 1/4 cup fresh peach juice and 2 tablespoons of honey. Leave on face and neck areas for 30 minutes. Remove with warm water, splash with cool water. Nice glow. Moisturize as usual.
Ingredients: Honey & fresh strawberries, papaya& peach.

Honey, Almond Oil & Egg Mask (hydrating)—Combine 2 tablespoons of honey, 3 drops of almond oil and 2 egg yolks. Put on face and neck areas for 30 minutes. Makes a good hydrator.

Remove with warm water, splash with cool water. Moisturize as usual.

Ingredients: Honey, almond oil & egg.

Peaches & Cream Evening Mask (exfoliates & increases the rate of new cell growth)—Combine the juice of 1 peach and 6 tablespoons of heavy cream. Put on face, neck and eye areas over night. In the morning wash off. Do this three time a week for a peaches and cream complexion. Moisturize as usual.

Ingredients: Fresh peach & heavy cream.

Rose Water & Jojoba Oil Evening Moisturizer (hydrating)—Combine 2 tablespoons of Rosewater and 2 tablespoons of Jojoba oil. Put the mixture on your face and neck areas over night at least twice a week. In the morning wash off. Moisturize as usual.

Ingredients: Rose water & jojoba oil.

Almond Oil & Lanolin Evening Moisturizer (hydrating moisturizer)—Combine 4 teaspoons of sweet almond oil, 2 tablespoons of lanolin then place the combined mixture in a bowl then heat in a microwave for 15 to 20 seconds. Add 2 tablespoons of water, and then mix thoroughly. Remove from the heat and cool then add 1 tablespoon of cod liver oil. When cool, place in refrigerator. Use nightly. In the morning wash off. Discard after 30 days.

Ingredients: Almond oil & lanolin.

Almond Oil, Cocoa Butter, Olive Oil & Vitamin E Nighttime Neck Cream (hydrating moisturizer) 2 tbs. Almond Oil, 3 tbs. Cocoa Butter, 2 tbs. Olive Oil (cosmetic olive oil) and 1 tbs. Vitamin E Oil or break open 2 Vitamin E capsule. Put the ingredients into a bowl and mix until blended, put the mixture into the microwave for 15 seconds or until warm. When warm, gently rub onto the neck area, front and back, in an upward and outward direction. This process should be performed in the evening before going to sleep. If you wish to accelerate the process, place a warm face cloth on the neck for approximately 2 to 3 minutes. Place the unused portion in an air tight container and keep the remaining portion in the refrigerator. Keep and use for up to 30 days.

Note: If you have oily skin or acne prone skin do not use.

Ingredients: Almond oil, cocoa butter, olive oil & vitamin E oil.

Mature Skin

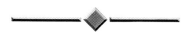

Mature skin is gradually being depleted of the elasticity, collagen and natural oils that once gave you that youthful complexion.

Some of the many homemade facial remedies are:

Sugar Cleaners (exfoliating)—After taking off your makeup and cleansing your skin, take a small amount of sugar, yes ordinary table sugar. Add a small amount of water. Rub the mixture on the face, eye and neck areas. This process will help to loosen

the dead skin cells on the very top layer of skin so that they come off easier. Rinse with warm water then splash on cool water, moisturize with your favorite moisturizer.
Ingredients: Sugar.

Almond Meal, Jojoba Oil, Honey & Peppermint & Lemon Oil Cleanser (exfoliating)—Combine 4 tablespoons or almond meal, 2 tablespoons or Jojoba oil, 3 tablespoons of honey 4 drops of Peppermint oil and 1 drop of lemon oil in a glass bowl. Combine and mix the ingredients thoroughly. After you have washed your face with warm water scrub your face with this exfoliating scrub. Rinse with cool water. Moisturize as usual.
Note: **This scrub is not for sensitive or dry skin.**
Ingredients: Almond meal, jojoba oil, honey, peppermint oil & lemon oil.

Sea Salt & Buttermilk Cleanser and/or Mask (exfoliating)— Add sea salt to buttermilk (paste like consistency) then put the mixture on the areas of your face that contain enlarged pores and massage for approximately 2 minutes. After cleansing with this combination use the remaining mixture as a mask and leave on for 10 minutes or longer. Then wash with warm water, splash with cool water. Moisturize as usual.
Ingredients: Sea salt & buttermilk.

Almond Meal Cleanser and/or Mask (exfoliating)—Combine almond meal with enough water for a paste like consistency put the mixture on your face and neck areas for 30 minutes. Then mix enough almond meal and water to wash your face, eye and

neck areas in a circular upward motion to remove any dead skin cells. Rinse with warm water, splash with cool water. Moisturize as usual.
Ingredients: Almond meal.

Baking Soda Cleanser and/or Mask (exfoliating)—Combine baking soda and water to cleanse your skin. After cleansing combine the baking soda and water making a paste, apply the mixture to your face and neck areas as a mask for 10 minutes to exfoliate. Remove with warm water, splash with cool water. Moisturize as usual.
Ingredients: Baking soda.

Olive Oil and Salt/Sugar Cleanser and/or Mask (exfoliating)— Place a tablespoon of salt or sugar in the palm of your hand then mix in some olive oil (cosmetic olive oil), just enough to make a paste. Rub the mixture into your face, neck and décolleté areas. Make sure that you rub this mixture in an upward circular motion. After approximately one-minute, let the mixture sit on those areas for approximately 30 minutes. Rub in once again then rinse off the remaining. Moisturize as usual.
Ingredients: Olive oil, salt & sugar.

Cucumber, Honey & Lemon Toner (complexion bright-ener)—Place 1 medium cucumber into a juicer then take that juice and place it into a glass container add 2 teaspoons of honey and the juice of ¼ lemon into the same container then shake ingredients until blended. Put the mixture onto a cotton ball then put the mixture onto your face and neck area. Leave

mixture on the face as your daily toner, then moisturize. You can leave this mixture in the refrigerator for approximately seven days.
Ingredients: Fresh cucumber & lemon & honey.

Tea Toner (lackluster skin)—Combine 1 decaffeinated organic green tea bag and 1 decaffeinated chamomile tea bag into one cup of boiling water. After 10 minutes remove the tea bags. Put the mixture into a spray bottle. Add one cup of cool water into the mixture and refrigerate. Use daily as a toner. Do not wash off. Discard after 2 weeks.
Contains powerful antioxidants to repair environmentally damaged skin.
Ingredients: Decaffeinated organic green tea & decaffeinated organic chamomile tea.

Honey & Almond Oil Mask (hydrating)—Combine 2 tablespoons of honey and 2 tablespoons of almond oil add the mixture to face and neck areas for 30 minutes. Remove with warm water, splash with cool water. For that luminescence look. Moisturize as usual.
Ingredients: Honey & almond oil.

Pineapple Mask (exfoliating)—Place a fresh pineapple into a juicer then put the juice on your face, neck and eye areas every 15 to 30 minutes. Remove with warm water, splash with cool water. Moisturize as usual.
Ingredients: Fresh pineapple.

Avocado & More Mask (boost your skin's collagen & fades imperfections)—Combine 1 avocado, 1 cooked carrot into a bowl whip into a smooth consistency then add 3 tablespoons of honey ½ cup of heavy cream and 1 beaten egg then blend all ingredients until smooth. Gently fold 1 drop of lemon oil and 1 drop of orange oil into the mixture. Place ½ of the ingredients onto the face and neck areas leave mask on for approximately 20 to 30 minutes, rinse with cool water. Place the remaining portion into refrigerator in an air tight container and use the remainder portion the next day but keep this mask no longer then 1 day in your refrigerator. This mask will boost your skin's collagen and will help fade imperfections. This combination should make two masks. You should always blend oils such as orange or lemon before using in any configuration. Never use nature oils directly onto the eye, face or neck areas.
Ingredients: Fresh avocado & carrot, honey, heavy cream, egg, lemon oil & orange oil.

Honey, Sweet Almond Oil and Oil of Rose Mask (hydrating)—Combine 4 tablespoons of honey, 4 tablespoons of sweet almond oil and 10 drops of essential oil of rose. Put the mixture on your face and neck areas for 30 minutes. Remove with warm water, splash with cool water. Moisturize as usual.
Ingredients: Honey, sweet almond oil & essential oil of rose.

Papaya Mask (exfoliating)—Put a pitted and peeled papaya in a juicer. Put the juice of your eye, face and neck areas for 30

minutes. Remove with warm water, splash with cool water. Sloughs off dead skin cells. Moisturize as usual.
Ingredients: Fresh papaya.

Vitamin E Oil, Yogurt, Honey & Lemon or Lime Mask (softens wrinkles)—Combine 1 tablespoon of Vitamin E oil, 2 teaspoons of plain yogurt, 1/2 teaspoon of honey and 1/2 teaspoon of lemon or lime juice. Put on your face and neck areas for 30 minutes. Rinse with warm water, splash with cool water. Softens wrinkles. Moisturize as usual.
Ingredients: Vitamin E oil, yogurt, honey & fresh lemon & lime.

Milk & Strawberry Mask (brightens dull skin)—Combine 1/2 cup of milk with the juice of 10 medium strawberries. Put the mixture on your face, eye and neck areas every 15 minutes for one hour. Rinse with warm water, splash with cool water. Brighten up dull-looking skin. Moisturize as usual.
Ingredients: Milk & fresh strawberries.

Tomato, Avocado and Lemon/Lime Mask (brightens dull complexion)—Blend ½ of a tomato, 1 avocado, ½ lemon and ½ lime. After removing the pit from the avocado, place the tomato and avocado in a juicer or blender until mixture is a smooth consistency. Empty the finished product into a bowl and add the juice of the lemon and lime until blended. Place the mask on your face and neck areas for approximately 10 to 30 minutes. This mask will brighten you complexion. Moisturize as usual.
Ingredients: Fresh tomato, avocado, lemon & lime.

Banana & Honey Mask (hydrating)—Mash a banana and add 2 tablespoons of honey. Mix to a smooth but not runny consistency, and then apply to face, neck and eye areas for 30 minutes. Remove with warm water, splash with cool water. Moisturize as usual.
Ingredients: Fresh banana & honey.

Apricot Mask (restores the skin's elasticity)—Put a pitted and peeled apricot in a juicer. Put the juice of your eye, neck and face areas for 30 minutes. Remove with warm water, splash with cool water. Restores the skin's elasticity. Moisturize as usual.
Ingredients: Fresh apricot.

Bael Fruit Extract & Honey Mask (improves skin's elasticity)—Combine 2 tablespoons of Bael fruit extract and 1 tablespoon of honey to your face, neck and eye areas for 30 minutes. Remove with warm water, splash with cool water. This combination improves the skin's elasticity. Moisturize as usual.
Ingredients: Bael fruit extract & honey.

Milk, Honey & Lemon Mask (exfoliating)—Combine 1 tablespoon of milk, 1 tablespoon of honey and 3 drops of lemon juice. Put on face, neck and eye areas every 15 minutes for one hour. Remove with warm water, splash with cool water. Moisturize as usual.
Ingredients: Milk, honey & lemon juice.

Avocado Mask (hydrating)—Mash or puree 1/2 of an avocado. Spread onto the face, neck and eye areas. Leave on for 20 to 30

minutes. Rinse with warm water, splash with cool water, then moisturize.
Ingredients: Fresh avocado.

Milk Mask (exfoliating)—Put whole milk on your face, neck and eye areas for 20 to 30 minutes. Rinse warm water, splash with cool water, then moisturize.
Ingredients: Milk.

Honey, Almond Oil & Egg Mask (softens the skin)—Combine 2 tablespoons of honey, 3 drops of almond oil and two egg yolks then place the mixture on face and neck areas for 30 minutes. Remove with warm water, splash with cool water. This mask softens the skin. Moisturize as usual.
Ingredients: Honey, almond oil & egg.

Egg Mask (tightens)—Use 1 egg white—slightly beaten with a fork, put on face, neck and eye areas. Leave on for 15 to 20 minutes. Rinse with warm water then splash with cool water before moisturizing. This process will temporarily tighten the skin.
Ingredients: Egg.

Pineapple, Papaya & Honey Mask (exfoliating and hydrating)—Combine 1 cup of fresh pineapple, 1/2 cup of fresh papaya, 2 tbs. of honey—puree papaya and pineapple then add honey. Mix ingredients together. Depending on your skin type, put on face and neck areas 5 minutes (oily skin) to 15 minutes

(dry or mature skin). Rinse with warm water, splash on cool water. Moisturize as usual.
Ingredients: Honey & fresh pineapple & papaya.

Lemon & Olive Oil Mask (hydrating)—Combine 1 tablespoon of lemon juice and 1 tablespoon of olive oil (cosmetic olive oil). Put on face and neck areas for 30 minutes. Remove with warn water, splash with cool water. Moisturize as usual.
Ingredients: Lemon & olive oil.

Banana Mask (hydrating)—Mash a banana then apply to face, neck and eye areas every 15 minutes for one hour. Remove with warm water, splash with cool water. Moisturize as usual.
Ingredients: Fresh banana.

Cream, Banana & Vitamin E Mask (hydrating)—Mix together, 1/4 cup of heavy whipping cream, 1 banana, peeled, and 1 vitamin E capsule or 1/4 teaspoon of vitamin E oil. Combine ingredients apply to face, neck and eye areas. Leave on for 30 minutes. Remove with warm water, splash with cool water. Moisturize as usual.
Ingredients: Heavy whipping cream, fresh banana & vitamin E oil.

Peach & Egg Mask (The AHAs in these fruits help soften wrinkles, sun spots, age spots, blemishes and can even unclog pores, egg will tighten)—Combine the juice of a peeled and pitted peach after it has gone through the juicer, add the white of one egg then beat until blended. Put onto face, neck and eye areas for 30 minutes. Remove with warm water, splash with cool water. Moisturize as usual.

Ingredients: Fresh peach & egg.

Peach Overnight Mask (AHAs will help soften wrinkles, sun spots, age spots, blemishes and can even unclog pores).—Peel a peach and gently massage the inside of the peach onto the face and neck areas every night for two weeks. Do not rub off. When you get up in the morning remove with warm water, splash with cool water. This treatment will completely cleanse the skin while cleaning the pores of all debris. Moisturize as usual.

Ingredients: Fresh peach.

Almond Oil & Lanolin Nighttime Moisturizer (hydrating)—Combine 4 teaspoons of sweet almond oil, 2 tablespoons of lanolin put into microwave. Then add 2 tablespoons of water mix well then add the 2 tablespoons of cod liver oil. When cool, place in refrigerator. Use nightly. Wash off in the morning. Moisturize as usual. Discard after 30 days.

Ingredients: Almond oil & lanolin.

Olive Oil, Wheat Germ Oil, Geranium Oil & Lemon Oil Nighttime Cream (hydrating)—Combine 6 tablespoons of olive oil (cosmetic olive oil), 6 tablespoons of wheat germ oil, 6 tablespoons of Geranium oil and 2 teaspoon of Lemon oil. Mix well. Apply nightly to face and neck each night for 30 days and you will see fewer lines and wrinkles. Hydrates the skin. Moisturize as usual.

Ingredients: Olive oil, wheat germ oil, geranium oil & lemon oil.

Rosewater, Jojoba Oil & Orange Oil Nighttime Moisturizer (hydrating)—Combine 2 tablespoons of Rosewater, 2 tablespoons of Jojoba oil and 2 tablespoons of Orange oil. Put the mixture on your face and neck areas over night at least twice a week. Wash off in the morning. Moisturize as usual.
Ingredients: Rosewater, jojoba oil & orange oil.

Almond Oil, Cocoa Butter, Geranium Oil and Vitamin E Nighttime Neck Cream (hydrating)—Combine 2 tbs. Almond Oil, 3 tbs. Cocoa Butter, 2 tbs. Olive Oil (cosmetic olive oil), 2 tbs. Geranium oil and 1 tbs. Vitamin E Oil or break open 2 Vitamin E capsule. Put the ingredients into a small bowl and mix until blended, put the mixture into the microwave for 15 seconds. When warm, gently rub onto the neck area, front and back, in an upward and outward direction. This process should be performed in the evening before going to sleep. If you wish to accelerate the process, place a warm face cloth on the neck for approximately 3 to 5 minutes. Place the unused portion in an air tight container and keep the remaining portion in the refrigerator. Leave on overnight. Wash off in the morning. Moisturize as usual.
Ingredients: Almond oil cocoa butter, olive oil, geranium oil & vitamin E oil.

Almond Oil, Lanolin and Coco Butter Nighttime Cream (hydrating)—Combine 8 tablespoons of almond oil 4 tablespoons of lanolin 4 tablespoons of cocoa butter. Melt of a low heat. Add 2 tablespoons of rosewater and 2 tablespoons of jojoba oil and 1 teaspoon of honey. Cool and mix until you have obtained a creamy consistency. Use mixture each night. Store in refrigerator for up to 30 days then discard. Moisturize as usual.

Ingredients: Almond oil, lanolin, coco butter, rosewater, jojoba oil and honey.

Peaches and Cream Nighttime Mask (exfoliates & increases the rate of new cell growth)—Combine the juice of 1 peach and 6 tablespoons of heavy cream. Put on face, neck and eye areas over night. Do this three time a week. For a peaches and cream complexion. Moisturize as usual.

Ingredients: Fresh peach & heavy cream.

Delicate/Sensitive Skin

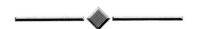

Delicate and/or sensitive skin does need special attention. Most delicate and/or sensitive skin types can use most products while in other cases, most products are prohibited. That just means that you, for the most part, will know exactly what your skin will and will not tolerate.

Some of the many homemade facial remedies are:

Honey, Almond Oil & Egg Mask (hydrating)—Combine 2 tablespoons of honey, 3 drops of almond oil and 2 egg yolks.

Put on face and neck areas for 30 minutes. Remove with warm water, splash with cool water. Moisturize as usual.
Ingredients: Honey, almond oil & egg.

Banana Mask (hydrating)—Mash a banana then apply to eye area every 15 minutes for one hour. Remove with warm water, splash with cool water. Moisturize as usual.
Ingredients: Fresh banana.

Cucumber, Milk & Rose Water Mask (whiting delicate skin)—Combine 1 tablespoon of cucumber juice and 1 tablespoon of milk and add a few drops of rose water. Put mixture on your face and neck areas. Leave on for 30 minutes. Remove with warm water, splash with cool water. Moisturize as usual.
Ingredients: Fresh cucumber, milk & rose water.

Banana & Honey Mask (hydrating)—Mash 1 medium banana with a fork then add 1 tablespoon of honey. Put the thoroughly mixed mixture on your face and neck areas for approximately 10 minutes. Rinse with warm water, splash with cool water. Moisturize as usual.
Ingredients: Fresh banana & honey.

Tea Mask (soothing)—Bring water to a boil. Add 4 chamomile tea bags to 2 cups of boiling water and let steep for 10 minutes. After the water has cooled, add 1 cup of cool water. Put mixture into a spray bottle. Use as a toner. Do not rinse off. Discard after 2 weeks.
Ingredients: Chamomile tea.

Cucumber, Milk & Egg Mask (tightening & exfoliating)—Combine the juice of 1/4 of a cucumber, 2 tablespoons of milk and 1 egg white. Put the mixture on your face, eye and neck areas for 30 minutes. Rinse with warm water, splash with cool water. Moisturize as usual.
Ingredients: Cucumber, milk & egg.

Egg & Oatmeal Mask (soothing & tightening)—Combine 1 egg white and enough oatmeal to make a paste. Put onto your face, neck and eye areas until the mixture hardens. Rinse with warm water, splash with cool water. Moisturize as usual.
Ingredients: Egg & oatmeal.

Milk-of-Magnesia Mask (firms and tightens)—Put milk-of-magnesia on your face, neck and eye areas, leave the milk-of-magnesia on these areas for 20 to 30 minutes. Firms and tightens. Rinse with warm water, then splash with cool water. Moisturize as usual.
Ingredients: Milk-of-Magnesia.

Banana & Honey Mask (hydrating)—Mash a banana and add 2 tablespoons of honey. Mix to a smooth but not runny consistency, and then apply to face, neck and eye areas for 30 minutes. Remove with warm water, splash with cool water. Moisturize as usual.
Ingredients: Fresh banana & honey.

Always keep in mind the sensitivity of your skin. Never put any product on your skin unless you have thoroughly tested it on an inconspicuous area at least 24 hour before applying to an entire area. Those of you with sensitive or delicate skin must be extremely careful.

Eye Remedies

Dark Circles—Gently massage the eye area starting at the outer corner of the eye and working your way toward the inner eye area with almond cream and wipe off after 5 to 10 minutes. Moisturize as usual.

Dark Circles—Massage milk around eyes for 3 to 5 minutes. Always working from the outer eye area toward the inner eye area. Moisturize as usual.
Ingredients: Milk.

Dark Circles—Massage a skin lightening cream very gently around the eye area for 3 to 5 minutes. Always working from the outer eye area toward the inner eye area. Moisturize as usual.
Ingredients: Cream.

Crepe-like skin—You can put odorless castor oil on that crepe-like shin under the eye area and you can also put the castor oil on the throat area. Or you can mix the castor oil with your favorite eye or neck cream. Leave on over night and wash off in the morning. Moisturize as usual.
Ingredients: Caster oil.

Puffy Eyes—Cucumber slices or potato slices or chamomile tea bags, put any of the above on the eye area for 15 to 20 minutes then remove and rinse with cool water. Chilled witch hazel, place the witch hazel on a cotton ball then apply to eye area. Do not remove. Moisturize as usual.
Ingredients: Fresh cucumber & potato & chamomile tea.

Dark Circles—Slice a fresh fig in half, place a half on each eye for 15 to 30 minutes. Rinse of. Moisturize as usual.
Ingredients: Fresh figs.

Reduce Swelling under eyes—brew a cup of rosehip tea with two bags. When the bags have cooled, place on your discolored under eye area for 30 minutes. Moisturize as usual.
Ingredients: Rosehip tea.

Bags or Dark Circles—Melon slices, place under the eye area for 15 to 20 minutes pat with cool water, never cold water. Or place melon in a juicer put the juice of the melon under the eye area before going to bed. Keep the leftover juice in an air tight container in the refrigerator for three days but no longer. Moisturize as usual.
Ingredients: Fresh melon.

Some fruits and vegetables contain different types of acids. They are as follow:

Malice acid: applesauce, cider vinegar and apples.

Lactic acid: powered skim milk, sour cream, buttermilk, yogurt, blackberries, tomatoes or regular milk.

Tartaric acid: grapes, grape juice, wine, cream of tarter.

Glycolic acid: sugar cane

Citric acid: limes, grapefruit, lemons and oranges.

Put one or a combination of the above listed ingredients on your face, neck and eye areas for as long as your skin type will tolerate the natural source of acid usually between 20 and 30 minutes. I use one or more in combination three times a week or more. Experiment, have fun!

Oils and Herbs

There are oils and herbs that can be beneficial to your complexion and they are as follows:

Rosemary oil and/or herb—stimulates circulation and tones the skin.

Rose petals—smoothes wrinkles, corrects oily skin, reduces large pores and improves overall skin tone.

Yarrow—corrects oily skin, reduces the size of enlarged pores

Evening Primrose oil—strengthens skin cells and boosts their moisture content.

Tea tree oil—will penetrate into the skin's cellular level. Adding one drop of oil to your favorite day or night cream will help moisturizer and smooth skin.

Above are just a few of the oils and herbs used today in skin care. There are so many it would be advisable for you to visit your health food or natural store, purchase any literature you can. Your computer may provide the necessary information you may need. Always keep in mind the research is up to you. You will be surprised at what you can make for a fraction of the cost and with no fillers added.

Please note those with skin prone to spider veins or broken capillaries should not use herbs or essential oils unless authorized by their physician. Those with Rosacea should also ask their physician before using and herbs or essential oils. Never ever use essential oils full-strength. If you use an essential oil directly on your skin you could irritate or even burn your skin.

Masks are a temporary remedy. If you want your skin to benefit from your efforts, please use masks on a consistent basis.

When using essential oils prepare a mixture of oils and combine with your favorite moisturizer. Experiment with your own mixtures.

It is by trial and error that you will find the perfect mixture of oils and/or herbs for your skin. If you have any allergies or if you have delicate or sensitive skin, please do a patch test first and wait 12 to 24 hours before using on your entire face, eye and neck areas.

There is one more home remedy that I tried and it an excellent one. I went to my local nursery and purchased an Aloe Vera plant because I had heard that this plant is good for hydration and this is what I learned.

Aloe Vera

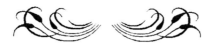

An Aloe Vera plant is a succulent that consists of 95% water and has anti-inflammatory properties. This plant will stimulate the fibroblasts to release collagen and elastin to make new tissue. The gel from the Aloe Vera plant is known to absorb into the skin's surface and penetrate deep into the skin's layers giving you optimal hydration. It will penetrate the cells and tissues like no other substance on earth. It will also clean the cells by taking out the toxins.

The Aloe Vera plant is the only plant that contains vitamin B12, minerals, amino acids, a natural form of salicylic acid, fatty acids and more.

I purchased two plants and I snip off one inch of the plant at a time and twice a day, I open one-half of the plant and rub the gel into may face, neck and eye areas. I do this in the morning and in the evening. One inch of the plant gives me all day hydration.

My hydration level has increased and my skin looks fresher and more radiant. I do recommend that you purchase this plant. The cost was $6.00 each and each plant should last me six to eight months. If you were to purchase pure aloe, it would cost a small fortune.

When you purchase Aloe vera gel and the cost is low, you are paying for the entire plant and not just the gel. When they pick Aloe Vera for cosmetic purposes, in most cases, they use the entire plant. The outside of the plant has no value but it is easier to use the whole plant and less costly for the manufacturer. Why spend a small fortune when you can buy the real thing, the plant, for partially nothing. Your cost is minimal, you know it is fresh and your results and tremendous.

14

Must Buy Kits

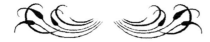

When purchasing skin care products it would be very cost efficient if you would purchase a kit. The kits should contain two, three or more items that when purchased separately, would cost a lot more. I find it very beneficial to purchase kits from skin care manufacturers that I would buy from anyway.

Some of the skin care kits I have purchased are as follows:

Murad (1-800-336-8723) or (www.murad.com)

The Murad II Advanced Performance System (#90205)
Your Kit Contains:
.25 oz. Eye Complex (SPF8), 4 oz. Age Spot and Pigment Lightening Gel, 1.4 oz. Combination Skin Formula, 1.4 oz. Night Reform, 1.4 oz. Cellular Serum, 120 tablets Youth Builder Collagen Supplements

Dry Skin—5 Step Package (#90101)
Your Kit Contains:
Moisture Rich Skin Cleanser, Hydrating Toner, Skin Smoothing Cream (SPF8), Eye Complex (SPF8), Perfecting Day Cream (SPF15), Daily Sunscreen (SPF15)

Oily Prone Skin—5 Step Package (#90102)
Your Kit Contains:
Refreshing Skin Cleanser, Clarifying Astringent, Oily Prone Skin Formula, Eye Complex (SPF8), Skin Perfecting Lotion, Daily Sunblock (SPF15)

Sensitive Skin—5 Step Package (#90104)
Your Kit Contains:
Moisture Rich Skin Cleanser, Hydrating Toner, Sensitive Skin Smoothing Cream, Eye Complex (SPF8), Skin Perfecting Lotion, Daily Sunblock (SPF15)

Normal/Combination—5 Step package (#90100)
Your Kit Contains:
Refreshing Skin Cleanser, Hydrating Toner, Combination Skin Formula, Eye Complex (SPF8), Skin Perfecting Lotion, Daily Sunblock (SPF15)

Murad Environmental Shield Vitamin C Infusion System
This kit provides immediate hydration while you help to revitalize damaged skin and to reverse the aging process. The Murad Environmental system includes: six 0.17 oz Vitamin C Infusion Treatments, six 0.13 fl oz Vitamin C Infusion

Treatment Gels with spatulas, a 1.0 fl oz SPF 15 Oil-Free Sunblock for face, a 0.25 oz Age Proof Eye Cream with SPF 15, a fan brush, and a 4-4¼" Diam. mixing tray. This system is an anti-aging and firming treatment, so you can start caring for yourself today by helping to reduce the appearance of fine lines and wrinkles while improving skin tone.

SilkSkin—California Cosmetics Corp.
For over 40 skin care: 3 step package
(SilkSkin Kit) Your kit contains:
Cleanser, Toner and Moisturizing Emollient
The quest for a complexion that is smooth and youthful begins with the SilkSkin System. This easy 5 minute program, infused with homeopathic remedies, vitamins and humectants, will keep your skin soft, supple and visibly line-free the way nature meant it to be.
(California Cosmetics Corp.)
(1-800 366-8243)

Lameto International" Skin Rejuvenation System (Entire Kit)
10 Aloe Enzyme Exfoliator, Hydrating Aloe Cleanser, Jojoba Bead Scrub, Replenishing Moisture Cream and Nature's Pearls. You will look years younger after you exfoliate the dead skin cells and hydrate your skin. After 10 weeks, this system will "de-age" the appearance of your skin reducing or removing lines, large pores, blotches, and acne scares while helping to restore that radiant youthful appearance.
This kit is for most skin types
(Lametco International)

Lametco International at P.O. Box 1240/Castle Rock, Co 80104 or (800) 933-2565 or FAX: 800-944-2565 or Email: Lametco@qwest.net

Joan Rivers—Results Kit
Contains Cosmederm-7™
The leading edge of skin care science and technology, packed into 7 formulas that work like mad to give you smoother, fresher, younger looking skin. There are formulas with Alpha Hydroxy Acids at levels high enough to really accomplish something, because they are buffered with Cosmederm-7™. Products include: Cleanser, Toner, Daily Improvement Treatment Formula, Eye Smoother, Nightly Improvement Treatment Formula, Exfoliating Scrub and other products. This skin care line will assist in the exfoliation of dead skin cells while giving you a more even skin tone and will reduce the appearance of fine lines and wrinkles
(Joan Rivers™) mild
(QVC) or (www.joanrivers.com)

Natural Advantage—Anti-Aging System—4 Piece Kit
This kit contains one 4 oz Daily cleansing gel, one 4 oz pore refining skin toner, (1) 2 oz All-day moisturizer and (1) 1 oz Nighttime renewal complex. Used morning and evening, the cleansing gel cleans while the refreshing refining toner removes excess dirt and oils without stripping the skin. All Day Moisture contains ingredients to moisturize and protest while its fruit acids remove dead skin cells. The Nighttime complex is specially formulated with MicroRelease technology to gradually

deliver Retinol to the skin in higher concentrations. This skin-care system can give you younger-looking skin in just one week. Within eight weeks, 100 percent of subjects in a clinical study saw a reduction in the appearance of the lines and wrinkles a decrease in pore size and a reduction of skin blotchiness or the improvement in the skin's tone and texture.
(Natural Advantage)
(QVC)mild)
or (1800-276-7102) or (www.naturaladvantage.com)

Principal Secret—Victoria Principal
An entire line of products for the face, neck, eye areas. This line also has products for the body, hair and an extensive cosmetic selection. This kit combines all the finest products from the original Principal Secret Spa line to bring you total skin care. It includes: 1 gentle deep cleanser (6 oz) 1 Time Release Moisture with SPF 8 (2 oz) 1 Gentle Exfoliating Scrub (4 oz) 1 Toning Masque (2 oz) 1 Booster Complex (1 oz) 1 Eye Relief Gel (.50 oz) and 1 intensive Serum (.50 oz). All the products work together to cleanse and exfoliate skin while also moisturizing and protecting it from the daily damage that can occur to your skin.
(All Skin Types)
(Principle Secret
c/o Guthy Renker, Dept CTJ
P.O. Box 57054 Irvine, CA 92618-7034)
1-800-545-5595) or (www.principalsecret.com)

Sellecca Solution

Sellecca Solution has a 90 day kit and if you order this kit you will automatically receive a Sellecca Solution club discount. This kit contains: Miracle Formula 1.7 oz., Facial Cleanser with Chamomile 6 oz. Bottle, Lite Moisturizer, Weightless Formula 2 oz. tube and the Critical Care Eye Cream .5 oz tube. Plus you will receive these bonus items absolutely free (with your first kit) Gravity Defying Eye Firming Gel .25 oz tube, Sellecca Shine Shampoo 2 oz., Sellecca Shine Conditioner 2 oz. and the Daily Facial Sunscreen SPF 21, UVA UVB protection 1 oz.

The Sellecca Solution skin care line is especially formulated for even the most sensitive of skin.

(All Skin Types)

(Sellecca Solution) (Connie Sellecca)

(www.selleccasolution.com) or 1800-655-4333)

Bare Escentuals 3 Piece Cush Skin Care Kit

Sea Soft, Sea Shine. Give your face a lift with this Bare Escentuals 3-piece Cush Skin Care kit. Made with natural ingredients from the sea, these nourishing, replenishing products are great for sensitive skin. The kit includes (1) 6.5 oz Deep Sea Foaming Seaweed Cleanser, a gel that combines deep pore cleansing and a soft. pH balanced skin treatment; (1) 6.5 oz Equilibrium Sea Facial Tonic, is a mild, yet effective facial toner suited for most skin types. Use in conjunction with a cleanser to help remove traces of oil and makeup that cling to the skin after rinsing; and (1) 2.1 oz Sea Life Nutritious Marine Moisturizer that's formulated to give your skin the proper care and to create a protective, moisture locking barrier.

(All Skin Types)
(Bare Escentuals)
(QVC)

Dr. Jeannette Graf, M.D. Recovery Skincare Set
Give your skin the complete pampering it deserves. This amazing set includes:
7 oz. Vita-Peptide protein Action Cleanser; .5 oz. Vita-Peptide Skin Energizing Boost (Mega-concentrated, provides a megaboost to the skin resulting in firmer-looking and invigorated skin; 2 oz. Vita-Peptide Moisture Release Treatment (Natural liquid crystals penetrate the surface of skin for enhanced release of moisture into the skin; 2 oz. Vita-Peptide Overnight Recovery Treatment (Enhances and reinforces the vitality of the skin by infusing Vita-Peptide with our fortified nighttime moisture delivery complex); 4 oz. Vita-Peptide Cooper Collagen Infusion(works with your skin's own collagen to firm skin); 2 oz. Skin Deep Wrinkle Treatment gel(helps reduce the appearance of dry, thinning skin and helps decrease the look of free radical damage around the eye area; 2 oz. Smart Skin Brightening Peel lotion (Contains AHAs and BHA's to exfoliate and sesame and mango oils to help keep the skin hydrated and smooth); 2 oz. Calm Down Anti-Itch Creme for irritated skin (contains soothing ingredients for the temporary relief of itching associated with minor skin irritation and inflammation)
(All Skin Types)
(Dr. Jeannette Graf, M.D.)
(Home Shopping Network)

Le Mirador 4 Piece Ultimate Firming Collection

Here are some essential items from the LeMirador line to help get your skin looking its firmest. The set includes these four full-size products (1) 6 oz Smoothing Glycolic Cleanser; (1) 0.33 oz Line Out Age-Erasing Serum; (1) 0.09 oz Firming Complex; and (1) 1.5 oz Performage. These four products will help lift and firm the skin
(All Skin Types)
(Le Mirador)
(QVC) or 1-800-345-1515 (www.lemiradorskincare.com)

Le Mirador Perfect Partners Firming Set

Beautiful looking skin is every woman's goal. Achieve your goal with the aid of the LeMirador Perfect Partners Firming Set. This set contains (1) 0.09 oz LeMirador Firming Complex Serum and (1) 1.5 oz Performage Age Defying Renewal Complex—a skin-care combination to help your skin look great. The firming Complex helps to tighten your skin and reduce the appearance of fine lines and wrinkles. Use the products together for maximum benefit.
(All Skin Types)
(Le Mirador)
(QVC) or 1-800-345-1515 (www.lemiradorskincare.com)

Le Mirador Day Lotion and Night Cream Duo

Give your skin the 24-hour protection it deserves with Triple-Action Revitalizing Moisturizer and Anti-Oxidant Night Cream. The day lotion is light, SPF15 has a UVA/UVB protection but a vitamin-enriched complex to intensively hydrate and

promote elasticity. The night cream promotes skin renewal and improves texture with the exfoliating action of alpha hydroxy acids.
(All Skin Types)
(Le Mirador)
(QVC) or 1-800-345-1515 (www.lemiradorskincare.com)

Diane Young—3-piece Basics Skin Care Kit
Start looking younger when you incorporate this three-piece system into your daily routine. Age Lift Hydrating Cleansing Milk, DeAging Firming Moisturizer with SPF 15 and Awaken Younger Night Cream. The hydrating nourishment of a milk cleanser leaves your skin feeling moist without that tight dry feeling. A night cream combines Chinese botanicals with modern technology to give your face a special treatment while you sleep. Last but not least, a firming moisturizer that helps to improve the appearance of line lines and increase skin firmness.
(Diane Young)
(QVC) or (www.dianeyoung.com)

Philosophy 5-piece skin care collection
(a must have) (Makeup is optional)
Makeup is optional. Great skin starts here with this collection of best selling skin care products from philosophy. The complete five-piece system helps clean, firm, and hydrate your skin—giving you a healthy glow without a touch of makeup. This kit contains:
8-oz. purity made simple one step facial cleanser; 1-oz. when hope is not enough facial firming serum; 2-oz hope in a jar

therapeutic moisturizer; 0.5-oz. hope in a jar eye and lip firm-ing cream; 2-oz. the present foundation clear makeup and skin perfecter.
(Philosophy)
(QVC) or (www.philosophy.com)

Hydron—5 Piece Skin care System

This five piece Hydron skin care system includes. Tri-Activating skin clarifer(Uncovers a brighter, more radiant complexion by enhancing your skin's natural renewal process with a non-irritat-ing blend of alpha, beta and poly hydroxy acids. Penetrates quickly, oil-free), facial moisturizer (SPF 15 Plus Avobenzone. Protection, today that helps prevent premature signs of aging tomorrow—with broad spectrum UVA/UVB sunscreens and antioxidant vitamins. Hydrates continuously, oil-free), line smoothing complex (Helps firm facial contours on application and softens the appearance of fine lines. Helps maintain skin's youthful-looking resilience and elasticity. Oil-free, ultra-hydrat-ing), eye moisturizer (Fights signs of aging where they show first—around your eyes. Reduces the appearance of fine lines and wrinkles after 1 week of daily use. Absorbs fast to ultra-hydrate delicate skin.)
(All Skin Types)
(Hydron Collection)(call 1-800-4HYDRON)(www.hydron.com)

Serious Skin Care Vitamin A Anytime/Anywhere

This kit contains:
1 0z. and 0.05 oz "A" Force Vitamin A Serum, diminishes the appearance of fine lines and wrinkles integrated with powerful

antioxidants Vitamins A and C to improve skin texture; 1 oz. One million IU's Vitamin A Cream and 2 oz. Two-Million IU's Cream designed to supply dry skin types with a mega-dose of moisture and antioxidants while aiding and reducing the appearance of fine lines and wrinkles; 8 oz. and 4 oz. Body Force uses Retinal Palmitate (Vitamin A) alpha hydroxy acids and other antioxidants to target areas of the body that are vulnerable to the visible signs of aging. The natural exfoliating properties smooth away rough, dull surface skin, removing dead skin cells to reveal fresh, polished, healthy-looking skin; 0.17 oz Vitamin A Moisture Stick—moisturizes and conditions creases and wrinkles to reduce their appearance, keeps lips smooth and supple, and can even be used across brow lines, frown lines and even neck lines. Hydrates and helps diminish the appearance of dry, wrinkled skin; 0.50 oz Pucker up Lip Slougher removes dry skin cells from lips and mouth area, providing softer, more kissable lips. Contains micro-exfoliating beads to maintain healthy looking lips, allowing lipstick to go on smoother without feathering. (Serious Skin Care)
(Home Shopping Network)

Serious Skin Care Retinol Magic Set
This kit contains:
(1) 5 0z. and (1) 1 oz. A-Force Serum concentrates on the visible signs of aging; (1) 1 oz. and (1) 2 oz. A-Cream Moisturizer helps moisturize the skin and smooth out the look of fine lines.; (1) 1 oz. and (1) 2 oz. A-Facial Mask helps gently exfoliate while removing dirt and makeup; (1) 3.5 oz. A-Soap Vitamin A cleansing bar; travel bag—black.

(Serious Skin Care)
(Home Shopping Network)

Serious Skin Care C-No Wrinkle Line Eliminator System
This kit contains:
C-Eye—anti-wrinkle formula rich in Vitamin C that moistur-izes as it reduces the appearance of wrinkles; C-Serum—rich in Vitamin C to moisturize skin. The colloidosomes, antioxidants, and botanicals aid are lessening the appearance of fine lines and wrinkles; C-Clean—natural and gentle cleanser removes impu-rities as it conditions skin. Enriched with Vitamin C and natu-ral botanicals, will help your skin be more vibrant and youthful looking; C-Mist—lightweight facial mist fortified with Vitamin C and aromatic oils, perfect for use throughout the day to refresh and energize skin; C-Cream—oil-free, creamy moistur-izer with SPF 15. Can be used on face, neck and body; C-Mask—cleansing and conditioning Vitamin C mask helps tighten skin, leaves skin feeling extra soft and smooth; Color Touch—3 concealer shades to hide all types of skin flaws. The creamy texture conceals naturally without looking made up. There is also a practical lip color.
(Serious Skin Care)
(Home Shopping Network)

Serious Skin Care Power "C" Collection
This kit contains:
1 oz. C-serum Vitamin C Conditioner—colloidosomes, antioxi-dants and botanicals help lessen the appearance of fine lines and wrinkles; 4 oz. C-clean Vitamin C Cleanser—a natural, gentle

cleanser that helps remove dirt and makeup while helping skin remain vibrant; 2 oz. C-cream Protective Moisturizer with SPF 15—use on your face, neck and body for sun protection and to help minimize the look of fine lines and wrinkles; 3.5 oz. C-soap Vitamin C Cleansing Body Bar—helps leave skin soft, clean and radiant; Black embossed vinyl tote is included.
(Serious Skin Care)
(Home Shopping Network)

Hydron 7—Piece Deluxe Kit
The skin care system is the most cost effective way to enjoy the beauty of Hydron skin care! This attractive collection contains seven basic full-sized Hydron cleansing, moisturizing, and treatment products, essential to healthy skin.

This kit contains:
Gentle Cleansing Cream 1 (6 oz. tube) Botanical Toner 1 (6.5 fl. Oz. bottle) Tri-Activating Skin Clarifier 1 (1 fl. Oz. bottle) Facial Moisturizer 1 (1.9 fl. Oz. pump) Moisture Balance Restorative 1 (2oz. jar) Fragile Eye Moisturizer 1 (.5oz. jar) All Over Moisturizer 1 (8fl. Oz. pump)
(All Skin Types)
(Hydron Collection) (1-800-4HYDRON) (www.hydron.com)

Hydron 12 Piece Deluxe Kit
The skin care system is the most cost effective way to enjoy the beauty of Hydron skin care! This attractive collection contains twelve basic full-sized Hydron cleansing, moisturizing, and treatment products, essential to healthy skin.

This kit contains:
Gentle Cleansing Cream 1 (6 oz. tube) Botanical Toner 1 (6.5 fl. oz. bottle) Tri-Activating Skin Clarifer 1 (1 fl. oz. bottle) Facial Moisturizer 1 (1.9 fl. oz. pump) Moisture Balance Restorative 1 (2oz. jar) Fragile Eye Moisturizer 1 (.5 oz. jar) All Over Moisturizer 1 (8fl. oz. pump) Tender Lip Care 2 (0.5 oz.) Botanical Body Polish 1 (6.0 fl. Oz.) Line Smoothing Complex 9 (0.5 fl. oz.) Micro-Exfoliating Cream 1 (3.6 oz.) 5-Minute Revitalizing Masque 1 (2.65 oz.
(All Skin Types)
(Hydron Collection) (1-800-4HYDRON) (www.hydron.com)

Principal Secret—Reclaim Your Youthful Beauty Skincare Kit
Revitalize your look with a lively glow. The Principal Secret Reclaim Your Youthful Beauty skin care system includes a 90-day supply of four fantastic products that work in tandem to help fight visible signs of aging. Each fragrance-free product is dermatologist and clinically tested. Specially formulated with Argireline molecular complex and HydaMoisture technology, the complete system indulges all skin types with essential moisture, aids in improving tone and texture, and encourages exfoliation. The result? Diminished appearance of fine lines and wrinkles for younger-looking, velvety-smooth skin you'll love to wear every day!

Kit Contains:
Total Facial Cleanser 1 (6 fl. oz.) Anti-aging Night Cream 1 (1-oz.) Anti-aging Day Cream with SPF 15 1 (1-oz.) EyeMazing

Refirming Eye Cream 1 (0.4 oz.) bonus Buffing Exfoliant 1 (2fl. oz.) bonus Youth Mask 1 (0.75 fl. oz.
(All Skin Types)
(Principle Secret
c/o Guthy Renker, Dept CTJ
P.O. Box 57054 Irvine, CA 92618-7034)
(1-800-545-5595) or (www.principalsecret.com)

Philosophy 2-piece peptide and vitamin c facial skin lift kit
Revive your skin! The philosophy two-piece peptide and vita-min C Lifting kit is an innovative, cutting-edge duo formulated for skin that has lost its tone, firmness, and radiance. It includes when hope is not enough lifting serum and hope and a prayer 99% convertible Vitamin C powder
(Philosophy)
(QVC) or www.philosophy.com

Principal Secret—Reclaim 4 piece Wrinkle Resolution Kit
Enjoy all of your favorite Principal Secret Reclaim products in one indulgent collection. Featuring the breakthrough Argireline complex, this comprehensive skincare routine helps to exfoliate and reduce the appearance of fine lines and wrinkles.

Kit Contains:
Total Facial Cleanser 1 (3 fl. oz.) Buffing Exfoliant 1 (2oz.) Anti-aging Day Cream with SPF 15 1 (0.5 oz.) Anti-aging Night Cream 1 (0.5 oz.)
(All Skin Types)
(Principle Secret

c/o Guthy Renker, Dept CTJ
P.O. Box 57054 Irvine, CA 92618-7034)
(1-800-545-5595) or (www.principalsecret.com)

Dr. Jeannette Graf—Skin Perfect Microdermabrasion System
Keeping your skin looking the way you want it is no easy task.
Be certain that you are using the right products to help you create the look you want with Dr. Graf's Skin Perfect system. This
in-home, deep-cleaning set is designed to help you reduce
uneven skin tones and roughness. It is a safe, effective affordable
treatment designed to help you renew your skin. The set
includes.
Facial Prep Cleanser 1 (4 oz.) Microdermabrasion Cream Peel 1
(2 oz.) Post Rinse 1 (4oz.) Night Revive Complex 1 (1.69 oz)
Over time, your skin will appear healthier and more youthful-
looking by reducing fine lines and wrinkles. This system will
give you a more toned, vibrant and younger-looking skin.
(Dr. Jeannette Graf)
(QVC)

Diane Young—3-piece Coneflower Skin Care Kit
A firm trio of beauty power, this effective kit offers three prod-
ucts for your eye, kip, and neck area. Maintain healthy skin
everyday! This kit contains: one 0.5 oz. Coneflower Eyeline
Firmer; one 0.5 fl. Oz. Coneflower Lipline Firmer; one 1.7 oz
Coneflower Neckline Firmer.
(Diane Young)
(QVC) or (www.dianeyoung.com)

Serious Skin Care Vitamin B Power Trio

Looking for help in recapturing that youthful looking glow that's now but a memory? Search no more—Serious Skin Care comes to the rescue with the B-Power line of beauty treatments. The Vitamin B Power Trio was created for our clients with dull, sallow skin tones that could use a new, revitalized look and feel. You also receive a sample size of the B-Illusion beauty treatment. Details of this beautifying kit include: 4.6 oz. B-Cold Flash—this Vitamin B micro-mist moisturizing facial water helps revitalize and cool your skin any time of the day or night. The special atomizer sprayer emits an ultra fine mist that won't interfere with your makeup. 1 oz. B-Surge—a Vitamin B invigorating facial serum that helps emphasizes your skin's own natural radiance. B-Surge helps your complexion appear vibrant and rosy and helps your skin feel refreshed. .036 oz. B-Illusion—this Vitamin B beauty treatment features a B vitamin and silica powder formula that quickly transforms into an emulsion on contact with your skin. B-Illusion quickly sinks into lines, wrinkles and enlarged pores, helping to create a smoother, younger-looking skin surface. 2 oz. B-Glow—a Vitamin B moisturizing complexion enhancer that helps give your skin an instant, fresh-faced glow. The Vitamin B complex helps condition and smooths the skin while the apricot tinted translucency complements all skin types by giving off a vibrant glow. Wear B-Glow under makeup to help banish dull, drab, colorless looking skin tones (Serious Skin Care Home) (Home Shopping Network)

Marilyn Miglin Perfect C 8-piece Set

Give your complexion, hair and body the beauty treatment they deserve. Marilyn's Perfect C Set features seven skin pampering products and a hair care product formulated with Vitamin C to help give you a soft, younger look from head to toes. This beautifying selection includes: 4 oz. Collagen C Cleanser to hydrate the skin; 8 oz. Collagen C Treatment Shampoo to gently clean and moisturize; 4.2 oz Perfect C Vitamin Cleansing Bar with orange Peel Extract this will cleanse and condition your skin with a citrus fragrance; 2.2 oz Perfect C Firming Creme will moisturize and firm your skin's appearance; .23 oz. Perfect C Plus this is a seven-day supply of firming facial treatment; .5 oz. Perfect C Firming Eye Crème which will diminish the appearance of fine lines around your delicate eye area; 8 oz. Perfect C Body Firming Cream this contains Vitamin C and Retinol that helps firm the look of skin and helps skin elasticity; .14 oz. Vitamin C lipstick This lipstick has a Vitamin C core to help moisturize and condition your lips.
(Marilyn Miglin)
(Home Shopping Network)

Note: The contents of a particular kit may vary from time-to-time one product may be substituted with another new and improved product. Always ask what the kit contains so that you are consumer informed. Some kits may be reconfigured to give you a wider selection or a new product may be introduced.

The above listed kits are made by some of the best manufacturers of skin care products on the market today. Take time out and call the companies and ask what kits are available and what kit or kits would be best for your particular needs. They will be happy to assist you.

If you have sensitive and/or delicate skin when you are purchasing a kit, mention the fact that you have sensitive and/or delicate skin so that the cosmetic representative can recommend the best products for your particular needs. Please be extra cautious when ordering any new skin care products and test a small area before applying to your eye, face or neck areas. An informed consumer is a satisfied consumer.

Skin care products do make a difference and will make a difference in your outward appearance. The proper skin care products will reduce your fine lines, diminish your wrinkles and even out your skin tone.

If you are consistently dedicated to the restoration of your skin with a strict routine of quality skin care products, you will take off five, ten or even more years from your outward appearance.

That does not mean that this process will take a lot of time, quite the contrary, when you select quality skin care products for your skin type and your skin's needs, the process is quite effortless.

It is very important for you to remember that you must exfoliate your skin to remove the outer most layer of skin. If your skin is damaged by the environment and time, you must have an exfoliation procedure. You must remove the accumulation of dead skin cells which give you an older appearance.

It is also very important to remember that hydration plays a very important role in a more youthful appearance. You must exfoliate and hydrate your skin with products made especially for your skin type.

When an informed consumer purchases a kit as opposed to one or two products, that consumer will save an enormous amount of money. Purchasing a kit is the most cost effective way to obtain skin care products.

If you are apprehensive about trying a new skin care line, don't be. If that product is not right for you after using it for a few weeks, send it back.

15

Conclusion

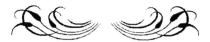

I would like to take this opportunity to once again thank you for purchasing my book. This book will save you time and money when purchasing skin care products and that is an exceptional combination. The moderately priced skin care products were tested for their unique anti-aging capabilities. The testing period I gave each and every skin care product would very from four to eight weeks. If a product did not perform as the manufacturer advertised that product was sent back and was not mentioned in this book.

I have combination skin, which is sometimes sensitive and dry a typical 60-year-old skin type that needed help. I was tired of buying skin care products that cost a small fortune and did not do what the manufacturer advertised so I decided to do some experimenting on my own.

You will not have to waste your money or your time ever again because I did the experimenting for you. All you have to do is to purchase some of the skin care products in this book, depending on what your skin care needs are and when you do, you will look younger and definitely feel better about yourself.

Most women want to slow down the signs of aging I know you do because you purchased my book.

There are skin care products on the market today that are treatments and those treatments can make a difference in your appearance. Skin care treatments do take time to reverse the signs of aging, so give them time, I did.

As you have probably notice that a few times in my book I mention skin care products more than once and that is because they work well in more than one category. If you can find one skin care product that works well in more than one category buy that product.

There are two beauty tips you should never forget and those tips are to exfoliate and hydrate your skin.

You must exfoliate to rid your skin of all the accumulated dead skin cells. After you have exfoliated your skin, you should hydrate with a moisturizer to plump up and lessen the appearance of your fine lines and wrinkles. It is a very important well-known fact that you should always avoid the sun. The time you spend in the sun today will accelerate the aging process in years to come. Instead, you can purchase one of the many self-tanning products on the market today. A self-tanning product will give that out-in-the sun look without doing permanent damage to your skin.

It is also important to know that you should spend some-time in the sun just not enough to damage your skin. It is a known fact that without the rays of the sun your body will not absorb enough of the Vitamins C & D. Without Vitamins C & D you will, in later years, develop osteoporosis. Just like anything else the sun should be taken in moderation.

I would like to see every woman enhance her own individual beauty so that she can look the best that she can. There is an old saying and that old saying is "if you look good, you will feel good." Every woman should look as youthful on the outside as she feels on the inside.

The society that we live in is more youth oriented than ever. I can change that perception and so can you. When you project confidence that confidence can be seen and felt by everyone you come in contact with on a daily basis. Most women have a business and a social life and in both, confidence can be seen and felt. If you have confidence in your appearance everyone around you will be able to sense that confidence.

The skin care routine and techniques that I mention are also needed. You must have a consistent skin care routine that you follow daily in order to achieve a healthier more youthful complexion. You will find when you get into a daily skin care routine that you will spend approximately 30 minutes from your facial exercises to your new skin care routine.

The descriptions I have given will help you select the skin care products for your particular needs. For example, if you want a temporary lift choose a product that says it will give you a temporary lift and if you want a product that contains Vitamin C choose a product that says it contains Vitamin C, and from that well, you get the idea.

Whatever your particular skin care needs, you will find the perfect product and/or products at an affordable price in this book.

There are products that are treatments and those products will take time, approximately four to six weeks, to repair environmentally damaged, line and wrinkled skin. After six weeks, you should be able to see a visible difference. If you are 40 years old it took you 40 years to look the way you look and if you are 50 years, it took you 50 years to look the way you look. It took time to damage your skin and it will take time to undo that damage. Your beauty transformation is not going to be instantaneous.

A good skin care routine with quality skin care products will definitely reverse the signs of aging. Taking years off you appearance can be very uplifting. When your outward appearance changes giving you a brighter more youthful appearance your mental attitude will change as well. When you look younger, you will feel and even be younger.

If you are in your 20's and 30's you can get a head start on slowing down the signs of aging. The sooner you start a quality skin care routine the better you will look when you are my age and older.

If you are purchasing this book and you are in your 20's and 30's, your skin care routine will differ. You will need a good cleanser and toner. Use serums and a good sunscreen. You too need quality skin care products and when you begin purchasing skin care products from this book, you will be purchasing the best possible products on the market today.

Always keep in mind that there are different skin types and that your skin care needs may not be the same as mine and for that reason, I have given you a detailed description regarding each product.

If you are not sure exactly what your skin care needs are, make an appointment with a dermatologist he or she can not only tell you what skin type you are but exactly what your skin care needs are. One visit with a dermatologist may be all you need and that visit is well worth your time and money. Seeking out an excellent dermatologist and knowing your skin type and your skin's needs will give you your new start toward a daily skin care routine.

Another reason for purchasing my book is that most of the products I selected were purchased from the convenience of my own home. To be able to buy quality skin care products from your home at a very affordable price is modern technology at work. Convenience and affordability are an unbeatable combination when purchasing quality skin care products.

I have found a perfect way to shop for quality skin care products and that way is via the television. I have bought skin care products from, in alphabetical order, Home Shopping Network (HSN) and (QVC) Quality, Value and Convenience.

The Home Shopping Network (HSN) and (QVC) are two television (cable) channels selling quality skin care products at very affordable prices. HSN and QVC are prefect examples of convenience and quality all wrapped up into one. If you do not get these particular channels, you can E-mail, call, write to them or you may go onto the internet. At the end of my book, I will give you all the necessary information needed to contact them.

Both HSN and QVC have a 30-day money back guarantee, which is almost, unheard of in today's skin care market. They stand behind all the quality skin care products you purchase from them. The skin care products mentioned in this book that you purchase from HSN or QVC are quality skin care products at an affordable price.

HSN and QVC both have skin care experts, quality control, which means that they are constantly testing skin care products for claims that are made by manufacturers. All claims made by a manufacturer or vender, must be substantiated by clinical trials. Absolutely no vendor and/or manufacturer of any skin care product can make any claim on the air unless that claim can be is supported by documented proof.

We, the consumer, do receive the benefits of all the testing made by the quality control persons at both HSN and QVC and those benefits are an unbeatable combination of convenience and quality skin care products at an affordability price.

Having a beautiful-healthy glow, with minimal wrinkles and lines and as little sagging as possible without surgery is what most woman want and if you are persistent and consistent, you will be able to achieve the ultimate youthful appearance at any age.

After you have chosen your new skin care products from your cleanser to your overnight cream, it will take approximately four to six week before you will see a visible difference. The difference you should see would include a suppler, softer and smoother complexion. Your complexion should appear revitalized and refreshed. You should also see a healthier glow; your skin should have a more even tone that should appear more hydrated. As I have stated earlier in my book, it will depend on the condition of your skin and how consistent you are in your daily skin care routine.

The products are in this book, products that will make a difference in the way you look. Look at the description that I have given you and find the perfect product for you and you will need a few but always start with a good cleanser. Your new beauty routine starts with a clean face and will end with a good night-time moisturizer.

The key to a younger complexion is to exfoliate. I exfoliate my face three times a week. Exfoliating three times a week may be too much for you and maybe you should start your new exfoliating process by exfoliating once a week. I found my comfort level and you have to find yours. If you go beyond your threshold of exfoliation, you may strip your skin of vital natural oils needed to protect your skin. Please ask your dermatologist for a professional opinion.

My dermatologist started me out with 30% acid for my peel and I graduated to 70% but no higher. Again, you have to find your own comfort level, I did.

I can speak for most women over the age of 40 and that is, that your lives, mature lives, do begin at 50, let's live it to our fullest capacity because we are worth it and we did earn it. Let's not let a youthful appearance be wasted on the young. You can have a more youthful appearance over the age of 40 you just have to work a little harder at what once came naturally.

Not all women were born with the attributes of a movie star but with healthy-glowing skin we can feel as though we were. Looking better will give you more confidence and that is what I want to do for you because when you look better, you feel better and so do I.

Contact Information

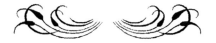

Home Shopping Network

Order Number:	1-800-284-3100
Customer Service:	1-800-284-3900
Product Inventory:	1-800-933-2887
Web Site:	(www.hsn.com)

Send Correspondence to:
Home Shopping Network
1 HSN Drive
St. Petersburg, FL 33729

Optional: Ask about HSN's own
credit card or their HSN Premier Visa
(1-800-284-3900)

QVC

Order Number:	1-800-345-1515
Customer Service:	1-800-367-9444
Product Finder:	1-800-345-2525
Web Site:	(www.iqvc.com)

Send all correspondence to:
QVC
1365 Enterprise Drive
West Chester, PA 19380

Optional:
Apply for the QCard Credit Card
Just call (1-800-367-9444) or (1-800-345-5788)

Credits

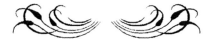

I would like to take this opportunity to thank the manufacturers of the skin care products and the beauty enhancing devices I have mentioned in my book for their commitment and dedication toward the development of quality skin care products and beauty enhancing devices which can assist in turning back the hands of time for all women who are committed in a quest toward a more youthful, healthy and glowing complexion.

Skin Care Manufacturers
Alphabetical Listing

The manufacturers of quality skin care products deserve recognition and I have used each and every product with success and I now wish to thank the best of the best. The manufacturers of the many skin care products, in alphabetical order are:

Almay
Alpha Hydrox
Bare Escentuals
California Cosmetics

Dermanew
Diane Young
Dr. Jeannette Graf
EcoGenics
Gly Derm
Hydron
Joan Rivers™
Kiss My Face
Lametco International
Le Mirador
Marilyn Miglin
Murad
Natural Advantage
Nivea
Olay
Parthena
Philosophy
Principal Secret
Sellecca Solution
Serious Skin Care
Sumbody

Alphabetical Order
Beauty Enhancing Devices

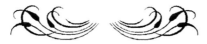

Beauty Enhancing Devices also deserve recognition and I have used each and every device with success and I now wish to thank the best of the best. The manufacturers of the beauty enhancing devices, in alphabetical order are:

Facial Flex Ultra
IGIA Therma Cleanse
Profile Toner
Rejuvenique Facial Toner

About the Author

At the age of 50, I went on a quest to find skin care products that would actually make a different in the way I looked. It was during my own quest that I did notice that other women were doing the same thing. They were looking for skin care products that deliver what the manufacturer promised and they were just as confused as I was as to what actually worked.

It was very frustrating for me when I went into the department store because of the variety of skin care product lines and manufacturers. Each and every manufacturer promised to do something from reducing fine lines or resurfacing your skin or reducing the dept of wrinkles. The frustrating part was when I would buy a product and the results were less then promised or nothing at all.

Additionally, when I would watch a commercial on television and that spokesperson promised a face lift in a bottle, I would but that product and again, without results. Some manufacturers are all hype and no results, it is very confusing. That is when my quest began for skin care products that actually did what the manufacturer promised and that is what I did.

I began to buy skin care products and when I got them home, I would test the claim by the manufacturer. If that product did what the manufacturer claimed it would do, I kept it and if it did not, I sent it back, if the manufacturer would send me a refund and if not, I just threw it away.

I did notice that there were many women that were just as confused as I was when it came to purchasing skin care product. One day a friend of mine asked me what skin care product would be best for and uneven skin tone? After telling her exactly what she should use, I got the idea of writing a book about skin care products that actually worked and here it is.

Each and ever skin care product in this book was purchased and tested by me for there anti-aging capabilities. While some are very mild, some will be very intense. That is why I give you a detailed description on each and every skin care product that I recommend.

All of the products in this book are for women over the age of 40 and for those of you, under the age of 40, please get an early start, you won't be sorry.

978-0-595-37327-7
0-595-37327-5

Printed in the United States
70768LV00005B/111